# Contents

# Preface

Writing a book about the system that turned my life around in dentistry never entered my mind. That is, until January 2018, when I found myself having a conversation with a very interesting and brilliant speaker, Mark LeBlanc.

We were sitting at a table during a break at the Jumpstart speakers meeting in Scottsdale, Arizona. The meeting was sponsored by Vanessa Emerson, the highly intelligent, driven organizer and founder of The Dental Speakers Bureau. There we gathered for several days and exchanged ideas to help launch our careers in speaking.

I happened to approach Mark at a table where he was sitting alone for a moment, and as we began to exchange conversation, he looked at me and abruptly said, "You have a story to tell. You need to write a book."

Well, that might have been the furthest thing from my mind, and literally took me off guard. My initial reaction was to say, "What do I have to write about, and what could I possibly write that could fill a book?"

Mark simply told me to gather some ideas on paper and we would talk later. By the time I left Arizona, I had purchased all of Mark's books, and on the flight home I read his latest, entitled *Never Be the Same*. The story and the title inspired me to look at my own life's experiences which ultimately left me never the same. I hope these ideas are also game-changers for you.

Robert Tripke, DMD
Chicago, Illinois
September 2018

# 1

# Why Insurance Dental Plans Are Not Your Friends

**F**rom one dentist to another: We are in an age in our profession in which the insurance industry is cutting off our very legs and thwarting our attempt to make a living commensurate with our level of education.

I have never been a participating member in dental plans. Why? Because they dictate what procedures I can offer my patients, and I will have to discount my fees to match those of the insurance company. I did *all* the work to get where I am, as did every other dentist. I didn't become a dentist for someone to tell me how to run my practice, how much money I can make, or how to diagnose and create a treatment plan for my patients. If that's the only game in town, then *I ain't playin'*.

The first dirty little secret in our profession is, we the dentists, own the bat and ball, not the insurance companies.

What percentage of your patients could you afford to lose before it would bankrupt you? 10 percent? 20 percent?

Well, I'm here to tell you that dental insurance companies are no different. They require enough *players* to field a *team*. If enough players stop showing up to play the game, then the game isn't going to be played. The dental plan coverage of today offers for all practical purposes the same coverage of *forty years ago*. Look it up. In the '60s, '70s, and '80s, good plans covered about $1,000-$1,500 worth of dentistry per year. That's right: $1,000-$1,500, in *non-inflation-adjusted dollars*.

In 1980, my crown fees were $220. That meant a patient could receive up to seven crowns per year under a dental plan. Today, a crown fee is at least $1,000, so the same plan covers just *one* crown per year. The cost of dentistry and the cost of doing quality dentistry have gone up significantly over the same time frame, but the coverage hasn't changed to allow the dentist to provide the same volume of work for a given patient. The average dentist not only can't charge the patient's insurance plan for virtually anything, but also are getting paid (as participating members) a smaller and smaller percentage of that plan's dollar.

I don't have a problem with anything a person makes in this country; if the market is such, more power to you. But I do have a problem with insurance company executives receiving a 12 percent annual pay increase at the expense of dentists and their staffs, who actually provide these services. Dentists give up the best years of their lives to learn dentistry, break their backs to provide patient care, and then are told as *doctors* that you can only see Mrs. X so many times per year and can only provide for her a certain number of procedures.

Sure, the insurance companies will tell you that you can treatment-plan anything, but what isn't being relayed is that the patients are being told, "If we don't pay for it, then it isn't a usual or customary procedure."

I realize I'm fighting city hall here, but I feel very confident that I speak for many of my colleagues about the problem.

There is a solution, however, which will be explored in the next chapter.

# 2

# Two Steps To Get Out Of The Mess

There are two steps to getting out of this mess for both dentists and dental practices.

The first step: Start removing yourself as participating members in those dental insurance plans you dislike the most (you know which ones they are). Do this slowly, over an extended period of time, explaining to your patients that as a participating member in their dental plan, you are extremely handcuffed regarding the types and quality of procedures that you can realistically even offer them. As a nonparticipating dentist, however, you will be able to offer them any procedures at any level, and they as patients will be allowed to make educated decisions as opposed to being told how limited their choices are.

I've also spent years educating my patients that, for example, at twenty-five dollars an hour in their job, their employer may be extracting as much as one dollar per hour to pay for their dental plan. If they run the numbers, that computes to about $2,000 per year in lost wages for the patient. That money, if saved each year, could provide a significant pool of resources for their dental needs (certainly more than their dental plan). Make twenty-six dollars per hour, bank the one dollar per hour, access two to four times the dental benefits (depending on the plan), and the *patient chooses* what gets done, not the insurance plan. Sounds too simple, but it is true.

The second step is to implement a structured periodontal therapy program and generate $300,000 to $400,000 per hygienist per year in a dental practice. I have been doing it since 1987: It's not a fluke.

## A Few Thoughts On Marketing

Marketing is something that for most of my years as a dentist was considered taboo. I built my practice, like many dentists, through word of mouth, which I still feel is the way to build the best practice. There is no question that a dental practice can be built faster (in terms of patient volume) with marketing, but I also believe a *quality* practice versus a *quantity* practice is done by word of mouth.

I had one experience with marketing in which I generated sixty-seven new patients in one month. For my practice, that was astounding, since prior to that push, I was averaging twelve to fifteen new patients per month. I offered a "complimentary exam and X-rays," knowing I would have to give something to get something. The breakdown on those sixty-seven patients was as follows: sixty-one wanted something for nothing, which, unfortunately, I gave them; five wanted reduced-rate extractions; one patient actually wanted to return to my office for ongoing dentistry.

Let me say, I'm not against marketing. If it works for you, then have at it. But I'm not selling merchandise. I'm not a retail store; rather, I am a provider of health care services. The idea of giving away services, to me, reduces the perceived value of those services, and says to the patient, "If they will give that away for free, what else can we get for free?" It sent the message that I need the patients; not that, because of what we do, they need our practice. How valuable are the services we offer if we give them away for free? Several of those patients actually asked how *cheap* were our caps? I felt like they were waiting for my Wednesday afternoon special.

## Try Ruffling Some Feathers

Fear of rejection is the big private-practice clinician killer. Dentists come by this very honestly. Too many dentists are concerned with being their patient's best friend, not wanting to ruffle anyone's feathers. This is where speaking taught me the importance of ruffling feathers, because ruffling feathers is how we gain case treatment acceptance. Telling the truth = ruffling feathers. You can't succeed by telling people what they want to hear, but only by telling them the truth. If that makes them my best friend, then so be it.

Too many dentists avoid treatment-planning anything, just to avoid rejection. I told my staff for years that I do not want to know if the patient even *has* insurance, let alone what type they have. If I am advised of this ahead of time, it surely will bias any treatment that I propose. For example, if I know a patient's insurance will *not* pay for crowns, that naturally pushes me away from those and into large restorations. This not only compromises that patient's treatment but is unethical.

I propose the correct and highest-quality solutions for each patient. If the patient wants to talk down the degree of quality, then that's on the patient, not on me. Rejection is your formula for success, because when you keep throwing quality treatment plans at the proverbial wall, sooner or later, some will stick.

The one single event that changed all of my concerns over patient rejection was the diagnosis and treatment planning of periodontal disease. In the 1980s, I didn't have the benefit of our current knowledge with regard to the oral-systemic connection: we did not yet know periodontal disease was linked to heart disease, stroke, diabetes, premature births, respiratory ailments, cancer, arthritis, and yes, even Alzheimer's disease. Despite this, I was receiving about a 90 percent case treatment acceptance from my adult patients.

The simple reason my acceptance rate was so high was that my patient education always started with the premise that this is a *disease*. There is no way to try and convince a patient that they have crown-and-bridge disease, implant disease, or orthodontic disease. But you can say they have periodontal disease. Disease is something no one wants to own. It is also a word that is seldom used in dental practices and needs to be, as it reflects the severity of a condition.

No patient wants to be referred to as a diseased human being. They will immediately say, "Can you cure this?" "Am I going to lose my teeth?" "Will I need dentures?" The instant that any one of these questions is asked, the patient has already accepted your treatment plan. And you haven't even told them what the cost will be, because they don't ask unless they want to fix the problem. And let me tell you, *they all ask.*

Periodontal disease is intimately tied to every procedure (except dentures) that you provide in the dental practice, and the ultimate success or failure of those procedures will completely depend upon the resolution and control of this disease.

There were two game-changers in my life that led to this breakthrough, as will be explained in the following chapters.

## The Power of Something So Simple

This is the story of Dr. Renee, a practicing dentist in Louisiana, who, along with his hygienist attended my seminar regarding the treatment of periodontal disease in the general dental practice.

Dr. Renee and his hygienist were in search of answers to issues both related and unrelated to dentistry. Little did I know at the time, but health issues and critical family needs were the primary reasons for their attendance. When they left the meeting, they appeared highly energized and excited about the potential for their practice.

Two years later, I returned to Louisiana and found them sitting quietly and reserved in the audience. As the presentation progressed, they asked if they could speak to the group for a moment.

What unfolded next was the difficult story of two people's lives and how periodontal therapy so positively altered those lives.

As they spoke, tears were in their eyes. Dr. Renee revealed his two-year battle with pancreatic cancer, which for those of you who do not know, is a *death sentence* upon diagnosis. His hygienist spoke of how the periodontal program had so positively altered their practice revenue streams, that she had been able to keep her job and care for her special-needs family member. As a result of this, Dr. Renee had also been able to keep his practice vital while fighting this terrible disease.

You could have heard a pin drop in that room. And there wasn't a dry eye in the place.

When the presentation ended, Dr. Renee found me waiting for my taxi, which was late. Knowing that I would miss my flight, Dr. Renee told me to put my bags in his truck, and he drove me to the airport.

Sadly, I was never to see Dr. Renee again, as he passed away, but he provided me with the most gratifying experience in my thirty years of speaking.

The idea that something so *simple* could do so much to positively influence people's lives has spurred me on for many subsequent years.

# 3

# My First Game-Changer

In October of 1987, I was in the private office of my new facility, and I was sorting through that day's mail when I came upon a flyer from a company named ProDentec (Professional Dental Technologies), and it caught my eye immediately.

Upon reading this flyer, I can still recall looking out the window of my office. The following words came out of my mouth: "Where in the hell has this been all of my life?" This piece of literature explained that lost revenue and inadequate patient treatment are caused by *not* treating periodontal disease in the general dental practice.

This was like getting hit in the head with a sledgehammer. My patient population was rampantly infested with periodontal disease, and I knew it. The problem was, I neither knew how, nor did I have the proper structural program to treat it and get paid for it. This, I knew, was my first and possibly only game-changer in dentistry.

You don't get more than one or two game-changers in life (regardless of what your business is). If you don't act upon these as they enter your life, you will, in all likelihood, never get another chance. I quickly grabbed the phone, called the 800 number, and asked that they send me everything I needed to offer periodontal disease treatment in my practice.

Three days later it arrived, and I felt like the kid in the movie *A Christmas Story*, Ralphie, about to open the gift containing the Red Ryder rifle. I opened the material and devoured it.

I went into my office the next day and probed all eight adults in hygiene, along with two of my own adult patients in restorative. I presented the information to my patients and spoke of the dental consequences (there were no other known consequences at the time) of not treating it. I received ten case treatment acceptances. That's right, *ten out of ten*. All were scheduled that day for periodontal therapy.

Now, I decided it might be a good idea if I informed the rest of my staff exactly what I was doing, because I wasn't going to wait to set up a staff meeting, I just did it myself. Upon later talking to the staff, they were all amazed at the ease with which I had gained acceptance and anxious to get on board. The implications were obvious to all of us; we had been neglecting this disease, and by treating it, would be greatly benefiting the patients and ourselves, as this treatment would obviously generate an entirely new stream of dental revenue.

I wasn't happy working in a mouth of bloody, red tissue and having to attempt to deal with it. My patient's teeth were being restored, but in a sea of blood and tissue that resembled a rare, uncooked steak begging to be tenderized. I was tired of the bloodbaths and the impossibility of keeping teeth dry for restorative procedures. I knew the only answer to this dilemma was to develop a structured system to treat this disease. I also was aware that all of my restorative work was a waste if placed in mouths like these, which would lead to total destruction. I needed to learn to properly code and treat this disease and to be profitable doing it. After all, I'm a very nice guy, and I'm all about helping people, but not at the expense of going broke.

We were off and running and never looked back. I can't imagine ever practicing dentistry again while treating bloody mouths and providing high-end restorative treatment to patients with a mouth full of infection. Interactions between our patients and the staff were so engaging that it gave real purpose to the dental check-up. Patients used to cancel or no-show at will, but once the periodontal programs were installed, all patients had an added incentive and significance to their hygiene appointments. They now knew the importance of both their numbers and their own contribution to controlling the disease.

Lo and behold, I then benefited from a second game-changer. I knew I could not let it pass me by.

# My Second Game-Changer

In late spring of 1988, my second life game-changer appeared, and it was a direct result of my first game-changer.

I received a phone call from the company, ProDentec, that had initially set me on the road to treating my perio patients. They had several questions for me, such as: How was I this successful with their program? How was I this successful in a town this size? What changes had I made in their program? And last, but not least, *would I consider speaking for them?*

As fast as that last question ended, I responded with an emphatic, *"No!"*

They asked why. I said I had no public speaking experience and I didn't think that getting up in front of a large group of people and talking was my idea of a good time.

They politely asked me to at least think about it. Over the next six weeks, I continued to receive phone calls. They were very persistent, and I continued to be noncommittal.

A few days later, a bouquet of flowers arrived at my office along with an envelope. My staff wondered who had sent the flowers, so I said to go ahead and open the envelope. They said, "There's a plane ticket in here." That's when I knew they were serious.

I flew down to Batesville, Arkansas, and had two days of conversations, then flew back with two carousels of slides. Today, that collection has grown into more than 500 slides as part of a PowerPoint presentation.

While in Batesville, I met an amazing man who over time became a mentor and father figure to me. Bill Evans was probably the most intelligent man I've ever known, and to my knowledge, he had a high school education. Bill was a risk-taker, and he took a large one with me. He took someone with no public speaking experience and allowed me, with all of my failures (and I had many) as a speaker, to develop my own style and pace as a presenter.

Bill used to call me after my presentations and say, "Tripke, you can't keep talking that way to these dentists; some are openly getting upset."

My response was, "Bill, I'm only telling them what is true, and I'm going to have to upset 10 percent of them to get the other 90 percent to figure this out."

One day in Cleveland I was speaking in front of a large gathering of dentists and staff, probably around 150 people. It was probably my fifth presentation, and ProDentec was trying to break me in slowly by sending another presenter to speak part of the day. At one point during my presentation, I said something provocative (as was my habit). My co-presenter, who was sitting in the back of the room, stood up, walked to the front of the room, stood next to me and said, "What Bob meant to say was…"

At that point, I looked out at the audience and said, "No, Bob said exactly what he meant to say and exactly how he meant to say it." That was the end of the apprenticeship.

Doug Billings, a representative of the company, with whom I traveled for most of twenty-five years, sat with me at lunch that day after the incident, called Bill, and said, "It's time to let the bird fly." I was on my own from that day on. I have been referred to as a "loose cannon" because I have never been concerned with how I make my point—just that I make it. (I don't rehearse my speech). I have always been extremely passionate as a speaker, and that is easy for me to do because the treatment of periodontal disease changes the lives of everyone involved. It's tied to everything we do in dentistry, and it is ultimately responsible for the success or failure of everything we do in dentistry. It permanently alters the outlook of every dental patient and the finances of every dentist responsible for treating it.

This, after all, is a book about a dentist and his patients whose life fortunes were turned upside down by the simple use of a periodontal probe.

On my way to providing my first seminar in September 1988, which was held in a midsized Iowa town, after landing at the airport, Doug and I got into a taxi, heading to the hotel. It was a miserably hot fall afternoon, and the driver was a lady with a parrot on her shoulder. She was dripping wet, as it was at least ninety-five degrees with 95 percent humidity and no air conditioning in the taxi. I still remember looking at Doug and saying, "If this is as good as this gets, I won't be around for a long ride."

Well, that was only the beginning, because the next day I found myself standing on a riser speaking to a group of about fifteen to twenty doctors. You really can't relate to this experience until you stand in front of a room of your peers with a set of slides as your only security blanket. It's a wonder I didn't soil myself. To add insult to injury, after about thirty minutes, it became apparent that one doctor in that room was there only for one reason; that was to challenge every word I said and to keep me as uncomfortable as possible. I felt as though I was a wounded man in shark-filled waters. When that day ended, I was drenched and ready to end my speaking career. Yet on the trip home, and over the next several days, something kept pushing me to go back and continue speaking.

I wasn't sure what it was, but I believed I had a message for dentists that was not only important but also critically imperative for their very survival. When I say survival, I am referring to their financial survival.

# 5

# Get Off The Rejection Merry-Go-Round

The greatest fear a dentist has regarding the diagnosis of periodontal disease is the fear of telling someone something they haven't been told before. The irony is that informing patients of their periodontal condition can be the turning point to disrupting the fear-of-rejection carousel.

Teaching people about a disease and the consequences of not treating it—not just dental consequences—then receiving acceptance and appreciation that the patients give back will do more to elevate your self-confidence and self-esteem than *anything* you can ever do in dentistry.

Your veneers are beautiful, but nobody's life expectancy is shortened without them. My self-esteem (and I didn't have much) grew exponentially when nearly every patient expressed the desire to have this disease controlled, and accepted my treatment plan immediately. As a result of this confidence booster, my subsequent restorative treatment plans were being accepted at a frantic pace.

People can *feel* your confidence or lack of it. The massive acceptance of periodontal proposals became the energy that propelled me into practice each day. The beautiful thing about all of this is I knew that, even in the most difficult of economic times, periodontal therapy was the staple that would always drive the economic engine of the practice.

## What Is Dental Success?

I have used the term *success* several times in the book already, and it is probably time that I define a successful dentist. (This will not include or address the *quality* of a dental practice because, for me, that is a given. There are *no* options for me to consider here: I will do it the right way, to the best of my own ability, or I won't do it at all. If I feel that a specialist can do something better, then I refer it.)

The color gray doesn't exist in my life (my wife and kids will vouch for this). It's either black or white, right or wrong, good or bad. There is no room for compromise. This is why *quality* does not enter my equation for success; it must already be present to even consider the practice successful.

In dentistry, I am assuming your work is already high *quality* or the *best effort you have,* so from that premise, we can move on. Success, as I have referred to it during my thirty years of speaking in dentistry, is all about financial freedom as you near the end of your dental career. By this, I am talking about the total freedom via zero dependencies on the government (Social Security, Medicare) for your well-being, plus, the ability to work because you want to, not because you have to.

As any dentist enters the twilight of a career, at age forty-five and up, stuff happens. The body doesn't feel the same, the energy levels are not the same, and inevitably, your ability to produce is not the same.

In 1987, my journey with periodontal therapy in my Chenoa, Illinois private practice marked the first time I had the pleasure of having *disposable income*. Prior to that, my life's vision covering the next thirty-five to forty years was that I would work until I was seventy or seventy-five. By then I hopefully would have retired my debt, could sell my house and practice, live in a nice rented condo, and watch the sun set until I passed away.

## First Things First: Debt And Investments

This may sound crazy, but that's exactly where I saw my career going because all I did was work to service debt. There was no light at the end of this tunnel. The debt never seemed to go away, and many days, it seemed to only get more oppressive.

As a result of my first game-changer (the flyer in the mail), my economic fortunes changed in ways I could only have dreamed about. My production was moving to levels that I could not comprehend. I was generating cash flow that I had previously thought was not only improbable but impossible. I was focused during this time on retiring my debt, and I mean laser-focused. That debt was going to be paid off before I purchased food to eat.

I'm sure many of you are raising your eyebrows, but please don't doubt me here. The debt was an obsession. I was adding $5,000 to

$10,000 a day to my practice (that's $10,000 to $20,000 adjusted for inflation today).

Coincidentally, at that time, I purchased and read a book titled *A Dentist's Guide to Financial Freedom* by John A. Wilde, D.D.S. I could quote numerous pearls derived from reading this book, but suffice it to say, the most compelling was the action statement stressed in the book, over and over again. *Retire your debt and invest your money.*

The key to investing is not just investing, but timely investing. The more frequently one invests money, the more productive the investment will be. For example, investing $50,000 on the final day of each year is not nearly as productive as investing the same $50,000, in regular increments of $10,000 throughout the year—meaning as fast as you get your hands on money, you should invest it. It will grow exponentially via compounded interest. This is a concept that many dentists, unfortunately, do not grasp, and as a result, the money either gets spent or invested in a lump sum, only to lose that compounded interest.

During this period, I would take any collections above my bills, and it was invested immediately. I was making three to four times my mortgage payments in order to expressly retire debt as soon as possible. The onset of periodontal therapy opened the door to massive amounts of cash running through a dental practice situated in the proverbial "middle of a cornfield." I retired, in today's dollars, $1,600,000 of debt in a period of only *two years*. Astounding!

I knew also that, historically, there has never been a ten-year period in which the stock market has lost money; therefore, I knew if my investments were timely, prudent, and diversified, they were in all likelihood going to continue to thrive over an extended period. Saving and investing became my mantra during those years because I was living in a time when the phrase "evaporating Social Security" was a part of the daily news cycle. I convinced myself that I would never be dependent on anyone or anything and that I wasn't going to waste the financial opportunities that periodontal therapy had given me.

# Any Dentist Can Milk The Cash Cow

You, too, can crack the code. You can solve the riddle. You can milk the cash cow. I happen to believe that *all* dentists are capable of doing what I did, and the *only* things stopping them are *not* implementing a structured periodontal program and the lack of discipline to invest those generated dollars.

I also believe that the structured periodontal program is the missing puzzle piece preventing dental school graduates from owning their own destiny rather than being obligated employees of corporate dentistry (more on the reasons many dentists feel the need to go this route in chapter 17). I feel most dentists intuitively aspire to be self-employed and employers, versus employees of heavy-handed corporate dentistry.

The periodontal therapy program, when properly implemented, is the ticket to avoid corporate dentistry. A single hygienist can routinely generate $300,000–$400,000 per year with this system in place. That alone would be sufficient additional income to service the debt of a start-up dental practice.

## Don't Ignore Periodontal Therapy

Unfortunately, most dental practices ignore the cash cow called periodontal therapy. Dentists are obsessed with the sexy and expensive toys of the dental profession, most of which do *not* meet any of my criteria for purchase:

- They don't make my job easier.

- They don't make my patient's experience any better.

- They aren't directly responsible for making me money.

Most dentists miss the most obvious source of care and income in their practice, which is periodontal therapy.

Many patients do not need crown and bridge, implant, orthodontic, or other such treatment plans. By contrast, virtually all adults need *and will treat* periodontal disease, and this is the first phase of any treatment plan that should be offered to a patient. Once educated and treated, most periodontally treated patients will adhere to the completion of the overall treatment plan, as periodontal therapy drives restorative treatment plan acceptance.

My goal is to help dentists see that periodontal therapy is their ticket to reach all of their personal and financial goals in dentistry. There may be more than one way to get to that destination, but nothing does more for the patient's well-being, the dental practice's finances, and the doctor's finances than a structured periodontal program.

Setting aside the benefits to patients, the purpose of a periodontal treatment system is to reduce the workload across the board for all employees and doctors while simultaneously doubling or tripling income. Who wouldn't want this?

## What's In Your Way?

One of the largest obstacles to starting a structured periodontal program is this statement: "We're going to think about this." This occurs all too often after a six-hour presentation. There is something called the *forgetting curve:* We forget 50 percent of a presentation within the first hour of its completion. We forget 70 percent in twenty-four hours and 90 percent by the end of the week.

Anything worth doing, then, had better get done quickly, or in all likelihood, it won't get done at all. The periodontal treatment program is successful in 100 percent of the offices that implement the system. The degree of success only varies with respect to how well an office adheres to the principles of that system.

I have been in offices, implemented the system, and learned within days that the probe is still *a foreign object*. If you can't take the first step, how do you win the race? The only way the structured periodontal program doesn't work is if you don't implement it.

Put the periodontal probe in the patient's mouth; that's where it belongs, not drawing dust on the tray setup. As my father always said, "You can't win if you don't play." Neither the dentist nor the practice can succeed if you're afraid of failure. Most people never get to live their dreams because they are too busy living their fears. Let me say this as simply as I can: people do not want a disease in any way, shape or form. When advised that they are in possession of a disease, they only want to get rid of it.

## The Simple Six-Step System

The system for treating periodontal disease is actually quite simple:

1. Inform the patient

2. Collect information and educate the patient

3. Control, but not cure

4. Ask the question

5. Make the appointment

6. Next patient, please

The adage *inform before you perform* applies here. The first step is to explain the periodontal exam and why it is necessary. What you tell the patient sounds like this:

> *Mrs. Smith, for years we have been observing and treating your periodontal condition, but we have seen over time that we are taking two steps forward and three steps back. As we have been slowly and progressively losing ground to this disease, we have taken it upon ourselves to become as educated as we can about the process. We, as an office, have spent a significant amount of time learning more about this disease and how to combat it. We*

*have developed and implemented a structured system that gives all of our patients the opportunity to arrest this disease process. The periodontal exam is the first step in identifying this disease. Here, we take a small ruler, called a periodontal probe, and record numbers that tell us the level of the bone loss around your teeth and the significance of any bleeding we might find. Both are indicators of active infection. As periodontal disease is one which destroys healthy gums and bone, it is something we want to control. This disease has also been linked to heart disease, stroke, diabetes, premature births, arthritis, Alzheimer's disease, and even cancer. The disease tends to reduce your body's immunity and thus makes the body more susceptible to contracting any disease. We will begin by taking a full mouth set of films that allow us to see the entire root and bone support of your teeth.*

Explain to the patient that the numbers will be read aloud and recorded. When reading the numbers, please be much more emphatic with the numbers that are four and higher. This is to bring the patient's attention to those *bad* numbers. Generally, before you are done with the periodontal exam, the patient will interrupt and ask, "What can we do about those bad numbers?"

Upon completion of the exam, reiterate exactly what the information means. For example, announce any bleeding points with the associated numbers such as, "Number two, distal-buccal, four, bleeding." By the time patients hear about fifty, eighty or 120 bleeding points, they will be wide-eyed and filled with concern, as they should. It is also important to allow patients the use of a hand-held mirror or intraoral camera to see the actual pocket and/or bleeding.

It is now time to have a conversation about the findings. The patient needs to understand the significance of these numbers and bleeding points. ("If I touched your hand with this probe with the same degree of force that I am using in your mouth, and it began to bleed, you would sprint to the nearest physician's office. Bleeding isn't normal in your mouth, either.")

By now, you have collected all the information, educated patients regarding the significance of those findings, and established the link systemically. Now you discuss the consequences of not treating it. Any questions patients may have are covered in our dialogue/sheet pack that contains the most asked questions and how to comfortably answer them, reproduced here in Appendix C.

The last step is to ask the obvious question: "How soon can we get you scheduled to begin the process of controlling this disease?" Remember not to use the word *cure*, because you can't cure periodontal disease, you can only control it, which leads to the discussion of maintenance. Tell the patient that this disease can only be controlled on a ninety-day (three-month) basis. This is the amount of time that daily missed bacteria—we all miss some—moves far enough under the gumline to perforate the tissue attachment, which is protecting the bone. The bacteria now begin to destroy the bone.

The patient is now positioned to understand the significance of every re-care visit. If the patient comes in every six months and is told, "Your teeth look great, no cavities, see you in six months," after a while, this is a broken record that repeats the same message over and over, into eternity. The patient begins to predict what you are going to say without ever showing up. So, my point is the repeated six-month dental visit message becomes less and less relevant to that patient. This is precisely why no-shows and cancellations in hygiene become so prevalent.

Instead, a periodontal therapy program offers the opportunity to escort the patient to the front desk and state, "Mrs. Smith would like to get started as soon as possible with her periodontal therapy." That's it! Now, once the operatory is ready, seat your next patient and repeat.

# 7

# Help Patients Control The Disease

Periodontal-structured hygiene maintenance visits allow the patient to properly control the disease and, in the event there are flare-ups (increased numbers or bleeding points), it is possible to immediately address those areas of the mouth, circumventing additional damage. This is nothing more than a race about who gets there first, the plaque or the dental team. When the patient shows up in a timely fashion for quarterly visits, it ensures that the patient, and the dental team, win the race. This ensures *no* further bone loss, and that's incentive.

I have often referred in my speaking to the reduction our profession has seen through the years in restorative needs (crowns, bridges, restorations). This is not only a real phenomenon but something we have inadvertently been responsible for. All actions have reactions, and many actions lead to unintended consequences.

In 1971, the number of decayed, missing, or filled permanent teeth per child between the ages of five and seventeen was 7.1. By 2004, thirty-three years later, that number had dropped almost seventy percent, to 2.1. In 2004 those kids are now thirty-eight to fifty years old. Guess what they don't need: Restorative treatment.

Dentistry is the only profession that does everything it can on a daily basis to deplete its own resources. Providing fluoride, sealants, and education to the population on a daily basis has severely reduced the need or demand for restorative dentistry. Before you overreact, I am not implying that these things are wrong. The use of fluoride, sealants, and education are precisely the correct way to care for our patients.

But there are industry consequences, and one most obvious is the reduced need for restorative dental services. My point here is, what better to do to compensate for those lost services than to begin treating a disease that is not only the number one cause of tooth loss but also has been linked to many other systemic disorders?

I'm asking you to continue your preventive efforts in restorative dentistry, but also to mine the true gold in your practice, which is periodontal therapy. There is enough *gold* in your practice's hygiene department to literally change your life or lifestyle overnight. If you simply exist off all other practice incomes, as you are doing now, and invest every dollar generated from periodontal therapy, I dare say that within five to seven years, you could be calculating your exit strategy from dentistry.

We all have procedures and patients that cause unnecessary stress to the doctor and the staff. For example, I am not a big fan of treating pedodontic patients who run circles around my chair while I am attempting to treat them. I am not the type to strap them in to accomplish the procedure. I also don't get excited over second molar endo; when I ask the patient to open wide, they give me a three-millimeter opening; and when I say, "Give me a big one," they give me four. Both these types of patients today and for many years have been automatic referrals in my practice. I now refer them from the reception room, as I don't have to put my hand in the fire to know it's going to burn. These patients need to be referred to someone with more patience and talent than I possess. I spent many years (too many) treating these patients because I needed the income, and I'm certain they took a few years off my life expectancy. Dealing with stressful patients ended when periodontal therapy began, because *I do not need* to treat them in order to financially succeed. That was *not true* before periodontal therapy became a part of my practice.

Haven't you ever wondered why a dentist has no desire to see the next day's schedule? Stress kills. Not just dentists, but all of us. My point is to get rid of it by simply weeding the garden. This is *not* an option, however, when every patient's generated dollars are so precious to the overall success of the practice. Once periodontal therapy arrives in a practice, those dollars become irrelevant and unnecessary and certainly not at the price of destroying one's nervous system.

## Finding My Way Back After Loss

Like all of us, my life has had its ups and downs, which they say builds character, but I'd rather skip some character, if you know what I mean. In 1978, while just starting my second year in dental school, I received a phone call from my mother. It felt like one of those "Where were you when this happened" calls. I was standing in the kitchen in my basement apartment, and my mother uttered the words, "Cindy was killed in a car accident." Cindy was my sister, one year older than me. She had been driving home from work in Carbondale, Illinois, and while trying to avoid hitting an animal, swerved and hit a large tree. She was killed instantly. I was speechless, shocked, overwhelmed, and devastated. The weight and reality of what I had just heard took me to the floor. I literally had no idea what to do. I knew the only right thing to do was to get home as fast as possible, and home was a five-and-a-half-hour drive away.

I remember getting home and finding family and friends all throughout the house, engaging in disbelieving conversation. I sat in the basement of my parents' home for two days and kept asking, "Why?" There were three kids in our family, and Cindy was by far the most creative of all. She had an amazing sense of humor. Someone once told her about a movie that had "grossed millions." Cindy's response was, "Geeze, I didn't think it was that bad."

The days leading up to the funeral and burial were painful and exhausting. We buried her in a yellow dress, one she loved, and went home to the emptiness that all families feel at times like these. I made a huge mistake when I left to return to dental school and hadn't given myself sufficient time to grieve. Dental school took on a life of its own and never really allowed me that opportunity. Cindy knew I was in dental school and knew how driven I was to succeed. I honestly felt I would let her down if I didn't push myself through this.

In 1997, my life began to unravel. I was going through a painful divorce from a woman who was my best friend and high school sweetheart.

I was involved in a court case for custody of my four-year-old son, which lasted two-and-a-half years. It was the fight of my life. It is very difficult for a man, regardless of the circumstances, to receive full custody of a child, but nevertheless, after nearly three years in court, I was awarded full custody. Bill, the owner of ProDentec, was very instrumental in me keeping my sanity throughout this process and helped me in ways I can't possibly measure. Without Bill's phone conversations during those years, I shudder to think where I would be. I will never be able to repay Bill for all of his help during that time.

My son traveled with me to every seminar (Bill made arrangements for this to work) until I was forced to enroll him in school. I always joked that Alex, my son, was getting a more well-rounded education with me on the road than he was ever going to get in school. Calamari and mussels became dietary staples for a traveling four- and five-year-old. Alex and I raised each other for nearly four years. Then, in 2000, I met my soulmate, Tiffany, who was a hygienist. (I always swore I'd never marry one). Little did I know she was a regular attendee at meetings I provided in Indianapolis. Her doctor used to tell her, "Tripke's in town. Wanna go?"

In 1998, I was giving a presentation in Indiana, and after the lunch break, I proceeded to start the afternoon session, in front of about 150 dentists, hygienists and staff. As I walked out into the audience, a voice kept talking to the point of being a distraction. It became so annoying that I looked to my right and said, "You'd better pay attention. We're going to have a quiz." As I said it, I noticed it was a conversation between a doctor and his hygienist. She kind of snarked at me as if I had embarrassed her. Long story short, I finished my presentation and returned home.

About two years later, I was in Memphis, Tennessee, to provide a seminar. It was about 4:00 p.m. on a Thursday, and I was getting ready to go out to dinner with the traveling representative from ProDentec. My cell phone rang in my room, and it was Doug, the person who normally traveled with me to a seminar location. Doug was in the office training outside sales representatives for the company. He told me he had met someone that day, a nice lady, and he thought I should give her a call; he thought we should meet. Well, me being me, I said, "How is that going to happen?."

He said, "Just call her."

I said, "Doug, you can get accused of sexual harassment by simply telling a lady that she looks nice in her dress. There's no way I'm calling her."

Well, I ended up calling her on a Monday night, just after I had put Alex to bed, about 8:00 p.m. We proceeded to talk until 10:00 p.m., and as I was about to hang up, I told her I needed to ask a question that was driving my curiosity crazy. I asked her if she had ever been called out by me at a seminar, and she said yes. She then told me that I had said "You'd better pay attention. We're going to have a quiz." At this point, I felt this relationship was probably now going nowhere! I proceeded to tell her what color her hair was, what she had been wearing and precisely where she had been sitting during the meeting. All this from something that happened over two years previous. Well, that obviously changed the vibe, because when I asked her if she would mind if I called her again, she replied, "I would look forward to that." This meeting of two people had to be preordained because no one would even believe this story.

That was October 2000, and we were married on February 16, 2002. At our wedding, Tiffany gave Alex a cross, as we were essentially all three married together, and she promised that he would always be her son. Alex went on (due to the aviation bug he picked up by traveling with me all those years) to receive his master's degree in aviation administration. Tiffany and I had one child together, and that was only by the grace of God. She experienced complications: preeclampsia. Things got so bad that the doctors told me at one point that this would likely come down to saving her or the baby, but not both. Brielle, our daughter, was born seven weeks early, thank God, *again*, and remained in the hospital for six additional weeks in an incubator. She wore a heart monitor for five months. We both slept each night with one eye open and one closed because if and when the monitor alarm went off, it signified that Brielle had stopped breathing and we needed to startle her to ensure that she continued to breathe. Today, at thirteen years old, Brielle is a sought-after ballerina prodigy who will be performing in Chicago regularly as of Fall, 2018. She is a straight-A student and competes nationally. I am extremely grateful for all the grace God has given me, and I count my blessings every day.

# The Cornerstone Of The Practice

The treatment of periodontal disease is the fundamental cornerstone of any dental practice. All procedures performed in dentistry are influenced by the patient's periodontal health or lack thereof. In that same vein, systemic health is directly tied to the periodontal condition of the patient.

Why a dentist would choose not to treat this disease, I have no clue. But if you're not going to treat it for the sake of your patients' dental health, then please treat it for the sake of their overall systemic health. We all have patients who don't care if they save their teeth (I have a few who don't care if I remove their upper central incisors), but none of us have patients who don't care how long they live. The diagnosis and treatment of periodontal disease receives a higher level of case acceptance and treatment than any service offered in dentistry. This, ironically, is how dentists can resolve their own fears of rejection, because a patient's rejection of a periodontal treatment plan is negligible. The only reason patients will reject this form of treatment is insufficient funds, but because of companies like CareCredit, the treatment is not only made affordable for the patient, but also profitable for the practice. Periodontal therapy and CareCredit were the perfect storm, as they were introduced into my practice at precisely the same time. Over a period of recent years, social media has played a huge role in patient retention, treatment plan acceptance, financing, and education. A company I have become closely acquainted with, RevenueWell, is extremely gifted in regard to all of these functions in the dental practice. Both of these companies (CareCredit and RevenueWell) are of enormous assistance to the dental practice in any and all of these facets.

There is a very obvious absence of oral hygiene activity both outside the dental office and within it. The reason we know this is that 75 to 90 percent of all adults have some form or another of periodontal disease, and less than 1 percent of hygiene services involve the treatment of periodontal disease. If you are looking for the missing link in dental services, then you have found it here.

When periodontal disease is allowed to flourish without any attempt to arrest it, then you are flooding the bloodstream, twenty-four hours a day, seven days a week, 365 days a year, with infection. Allowing this to occur over a period of ten, twenty, or more years make it highly improbable or impossible for systemic health to be sustained. Something inevitably will take a hit, whether it's the heart, lungs, brain, joints, or a blood-borne disorder (diabetes, cancer). A person's body simply can't tolerate an IV of infection to that level and to that extent.

The time-tested system for the implementation of a periodontal program is nearly flawless, and eliminates the following dental practice concerns: quality of service provided, financial issues, busyness problems, excessive working hours, stressful dental procedures, legal implications, and more.

## Making Periodontal Disease Real For The Most Resistant Of Patients

In thirty years of presenting periodontal treatment plans, I've encountered only one patient who, regardless of what I had to say, couldn't be convinced of his diseased condition. This man was not a gingivitis patient, but rather a type III (moderate chronic periodontal disease) patient. I became so frustrated with him that I left the hygiene treatment room and went to the kitchen in my office, where I grabbed a cracker. I then returned to the hygiene room with the cracker in hand, and I grabbed a cleoid off the tray and proceeded to load the cracker (out of his mouth) with plaque, calculus, blood, and pus. I then held the cracker out for him and said, "eat it." He responded, "Gross!" So I said, "What's gross? I came in here with a clean cracker. Who ruined it?"

I proceeded to tell him that each time he consumed a Big Mac, Wendy's burger, or Pizza Hut pizza, he was chewing it, swallowing it, and loving it, unless he was puking after every bite. The moral to this story is that, if they eat the cracker, then you send them home, it's truly hopeless. Oh, and one more point: Don't use the cracker technique on all your patients. Save it for the special ones. You will know who they are.

## On Insurance And Treatment Delays

With respect to dental insurance, I have *never* predetermined any dental procedure in *my* practice. One reason is that I don't have to, because in 94 percent of all (nonparticipating) policies it is not a requirement. The second reason is that as the patient is treatment planned, the urgency of treatment is stressed. Now, if insurance drives treatment, that same patient walks to the front desk and is told, "We will submit this to your insurance company and as soon as we get permission, we will notify you." The patient has just received two conflicting statements: One says, "Urgent," and the other says, "Wait." The control over that treatment has been relinquished to the insurance company. That's *not a good thing*. The insurance company can now drag their feet for as long as they wish (sometimes three, five, six weeks); the longer they drag them, the more money they generate in interest, because the longer those premium payments sit in their bank accounts, the more money they make. And while some people may think we are talking "only" about a $1,000 treatment plan, that's simply not true. We are dealing with an insurance company that has twenty million of those treatment plans backlogged. Delaying treatment (and payment) for each represents an enormous amount of interest revenue.

When the patient is finally notified that the insurance company has "given their permission" and you call that patient to schedule treatment, their first thought is, "If you can leave me out here waiting for that long, then how urgent can it be?"

So, you can see how the insurance cycle is likely to end. No dental work completed, no money, no patient improvement, and then, when they reappear at their next hygiene visit, the same cycle of events is repeated. This is how dental offices fail, not succeed. Predetermination is how you, Doctor, predetermine that none of your treatment is ever accepted or paid for. This sequence of events is not an accident; rather, it's by design—a result of clever thinking and a backdoor way of making enormous amounts of money by insurance companies. The office loses, the patient loses, and the insurance company takes the prize.

I maintain that it is important to educate patients that insurance companies are *not* in business to provide high-quality solutions for them, but to make money. That is *all* they are in business to do. The dental practice, however, is in business to do what's legally, morally, and ethically right for the patient, and *also* to *ethically* generate a profit. A dental practice can't provide quality services without generating a profit because you're too busy cutting corners.

## Is Your Prophy Business Earning Or Losing Money?

Prophylaxis (prophy) is a misunderstood term in dentistry and, as a result, is the single most expensive mistake a dental office makes. Until an office properly defines a prophy service, there is no hope of establishing or succeeding with the structured periodontal program.

In its most basic form, a prophy represents that which is treated *above* the gumline, whereas periodontal therapy is that which is treated below the gumline. How can you treat a disease that exists *below* the gumline by providing so-called therapy (prophy) *above* the gumline?

One of the most glaring mistakes occurring in most (more than 80 percent) dental practices is administering therapeutic procedures during a nontherapeutic visit. In other words, scaling and root planning are occurring during the prophy visit. To add insult to injury, the patient isn't charged for it, nor can they be. If scaling and root planning occur during the prophy, then it's free. The insurance company will *not* pay for both; instead, it will reimburse for the cheapest of the two provided services. In this case, that is the prophylaxis. Distinguishing between these services is what is preventing your office from collecting an additional $300,000-$400,000 per year per hygienist. The definition of a prophy is, even in layman's terms, extremely simple, yet for some obscure reason, tends to be missed by most dental practices.

Doug Billings, who traveled with me for twenty-five years during my speaking career, has been given an ultimatum: he must outlive me! He is responsible for the four words that will go on my gravestone: "They never got it." Those words refer to any and all dentists that I had the pleasure of speaking to that unfortunately, *never* grasped this concept. It truly is one of the most frustrating ordeals of my lifetime. This system solves *every* possible issue that a dental office can encounter.

In September of 1988, when I began the speaking journey that has now lasted thirty years, I honestly felt that the concept of treating periodontal disease was so obvious, so beneficial to the patient and the practice, that my speaking career would last only about two years. This is about how much time I thought it would require for the majority of the country's dentists to figure this issue out. Word of mouth *alone* should have achieved the task, let alone educational seminars. But no;

we are now thirty years removed, and still, more than 80 percent of all American hygiene departments are costing the practice money.

If you doubt the veracity of this, then write down what you pay your hygienist per hour. It's irrelevant whether they are paid hourly, are salaried, commissioned, or bonused. The hygienist is payed X dollars per month and they work X hours per month. Divide one by the other and you've got the hourly rate. But this isn't the *only* cost of the hygienist. Add in the costs of Social Security, Unemployment insurance, pension and profit sharing; and yes, some of us even pay for health care costs. This still isn't the full cost of the hygienist; sterilizations costs, if you have met every OSHA standard there is, is costing more than $20 per hour in that operatory. And we *still* haven't covered all the costs, because there are materials used in the operatory and the cost per hour to make the payments on the chairs that the doctor, hygienist and patient sit in.

Now, total all those costs and compare it to what you charge the patient for forty-five to sixty minutes. It will become obvious that the practice has lost its proverbial shorts.

Thirty, forty, and fifty years ago, hygiene was labeled a "loss leader," but that wasn't a problem then, because back then, at the end of every hygiene visit, the doctor received a bunch of restorative dentistry work. Where has the focus been in our industry over the last twenty-five to thirty years? *Prevention.* We fluoride, seal, and educate everyone in sight. Then we go home at night, scratch our collective heads, and ask, "Where did the restorative go?" I'll tell you where it went: You got rid of it.

This is the *only* profession I am aware of that does *everything* it can on a daily basis to slit its own throat, and I'm *not* telling you that what you're doing is wrong. It isn't. I am asking you to wake up, smell the coffee, and begin to realize that if you're going to deplete one part of our profession (restorative work) by doing the right thing, then you had better do something to compensate for the loss.

What better thing can you do than to begin treating a disease that is not only the number one cause of tooth loss, but has been linked to so many other systemic disorders, not the least of which is shortening the human life expectancy?

Dentistry has spent thirty to forty years depleting its own resources— the unintended consequence of doing what is *right* for the patients. As stated previously, by the late 70s and into the 80s, the focus in dentistry moved to prevention of cavities, *not* periodontal disease. Eighty percent of the adult United States population has mild to moderate periodontal disease, and 90 percent of the adults ages fifty-five to sixty-four have moderate to severe periodontal disease. If 80 percent had mild to moderate cavities and 90 percent had moderate to severe cavities, this profession would be in hog heaven treating decay. I don't know too many instances in which a cavity shortened someone's life expectancy.

The primary future source of dental income will involve patients forty-five years of age and up. The dentist who grasps these statistics and capitalizes on the treatment of periodontal disease will be the envy of his/her colleagues in regard to financial stability. The fact that restorative dentistry has dropped precipitously over the last twenty to thirty years simply means that the very financial survival of a dental practice depends on the treatment of this disease.

## A Word About Lawsuits

Finally, the legal ramifications of *not* treating periodontal disease need also to be addressed. We live in a very litigious society, one in which people seem to look for ways and reasons to sue someone. The best defense against a lawsuit is to do what is necessary to prevent one. Dentists are usually sued for one of two reasons: Either they did something wrong, or they failed to do anything at all. Both of these apply to the treatment or lack thereof of periodontal disease. Without question, your records are your best defense, because the courts seldom have interest in hearing input from your staff.

Several steps involved in preventing a lawsuit include:

- Thoroughly documenting all periodontal findings (pocket depth, recession, bleeding points, and attachment position)

- Taking six recorded measurements (DB, B, MB, ML, L, DL) at every hygiene visit unless periodontal therapy is taking place

- Always providing the highest of quality care, not just settling for the standard of care

- Telling your patient the truth, not just what they want to hear Being your patient's best friend cannot be your primary objective, or you are destined to be financially strapped your entire life as a dentist. I have countless friends in the dental profession whose sole purpose of existence is "not to ruffle anyone's feathers." If you're not ruffling anyone's feathers, then you're not telling the truth, and if you're not telling the truth, then you're cheating yourself and your patients.

- Making appropriate referrals
  When, on occasion, a patient refuses your treatment plan, then refer the patient to a specialist. One I consulted for has a dental practice that sits adjacent to the periodontist's office. I suggested that if a patient refuses treatment, I would personally escort the patient to the periodontist's front desk.

- Last but not least, having patients sign a treatment refusal form. The fact that this document is signed doesn't mean they can't say later that they were "unaware" of what they were signing, but, with all these boxes checked, you should have sufficient ammunition to mount a respectable case in court.

The periodontal program guarantees your hygienist sufficient time to educate, answer questions, and simply have conversation with the patient without feeling rushed. There is also more than enough time to provide the therapy because you, the hygienist, control all of your timeframes. Whether you need an hour per quadrant to treat the patient or a specific quadrant requires two hours, the hygienists always control their own destiny. The fee for all periodontal therapy is, and should be, based on the amount of time needed to treat that patient. No one in the office dictates to the doctor the amount of time he/she will be given to provide restorative dentistry. By the same token, no one will dictate those time frames for the hygienists either. This way, the hygienists never find themselves boxed in with insufficient time, and if they do, then they can simply look in the mirror. This is precisely the reason that it is nearly impossible for a hygienist once involved in a structured periodontal program to ever return to the "bloody prophy mill." Once you've tasted steak it's very difficult to return to a steady diet of hamburger.

## Empowering Hygienists, Building Restorative Production

I have never met a hygienist who cannot perform periodontal therapy, but I have seen countless situations in which the hygienist is doing it, the doctor isn't getting paid for it, and the hygienist doesn't have enough time to treat the patient. If you ask the hygienists what their chief complaint is, inside the walls of a dental office, their response will be, "I don't have enough time to treat my patient."

The reason is that virtually every dentist blocks the same amount of time for every patient that sits in the hygiene chair. Some of those should and could be out of that chair in twenty-two minutes, while others could justify eight hours per quadrant scaling and root planning. The problem here is that the hygienist gets boxed into a corner, forced to decide whether to excuse the patient after the allotted time, leaving the sub (-calculus, -plaque, etc.) under the gumline, knowing the job wasn't completed correctly, or to keep the patient in the chair, remove the subgingival debris, and fall forty-five to sixty minutes behind on the schedule.

At this point, you know who is looking over the hygienist's shoulder. You see, it doesn't matter which of these two options the hygienist chooses: It's a lose-lose.

The dentist feels responsible for establishing time restrictions on the hygienist. This is your first mistake; doctors are not providing treatment and have literally no idea the time required to obtain periodontal health in the mouth of any patient. Only the person providing that treatment truly knows the time needed to accomplish periodontal health. Most commonly, forty-five to sixty minutes are blocked to collect information (exams and radiographs), formulate a treatment plan, make all the necessary assessments, and still treat the patient. A disease cannot be diagnosed, treatment planned, and treated in forty-five to sixty minutes. That's impossible. Every patient is also obviously different and therefore the time needed will vary from patient to patient.

Long before intraoral cameras were in vogue, the treatment of periodontal disease was the driving force in the case treatment acceptance of restorative care. During a hygiene visit, both the dentist and hygienist stress the urgency of treatment for a fractured cusp, broken restoration, or recurrent decay, for example. But the patient's most common response is, "Well it doesn't hurt." Here's the beautiful thing about periodontal disease: It doesn't hurt, either.

Pain as part of periodontal disease generally means it's "four on the floor" as the teeth are coming out. But despite no pain, the patient still learns in treating their periodontal condition that the mouth will smell better, look better, taste better, and feel better, despite the fact that there was no pain. Through this exercise, the patient learns that pain is not a prerequisite for needing dental treatment. This learning process occurs naturally and directly begins to accelerate restorative acceptance in the practice.

Due to tremendous success in providing periodontal therapy, my patients' confidence in me as a provider also grew exponentially. These are the precise reasons that my restorative case treatment acceptance exploded. During the first four years of the periodontal program, I was averaging six to ten units of crown and bridge per day. One day that I distinctly remember was a day in which I produced seventeen units of crown and bridge. At the end of that day I was found lying on my back in an unequipped treatment room. My hygienist walked by and said, "What's your problem?" and I replied, "I'm exhausted." At that point, my receptionist walked by and said, "Well, you might as well get used to it. Tomorrow is no different." I was literally dumbfounded that seemingly endless, highly productive days were caused by teaching people about periodontal disease, but that was exactly what ignited my practice. No consultant or magic strategy taught me to "gain case treatment acceptance." No; it was simply educating the patient about a disease, and the rest was history.

I am commonly asked by meeting planners about problems in the dental profession that are associated with the influx of corporate dentistry. My answer to *all* issues to corporate influx is: "Diagnose and treat periodontal disease." The reason that dentists and dental school graduates feel an obligation to enter corporate, is they seemingly have no way to service their own debt (which averages $280,000–$480,000, and that's before dentists even consider buying an existing practice or building one of their own—more on that in chapter 17). The math just doesn't compute, and I completely understand. For just a moment, however, imagine adding $300,000–$400,000 per year per hygienist to the income of a dental practice, and then try to explain why *anyone* has to enter corporate dentistry. The treatment of periodontal disease and its ability to create generational wealth while doing what is right for the patient is *the* answer to corporate issues.

## The Oral-Systemic Connection

The connection between physicians and dentists has never been more apparent or obvious, due to the systemic links between periodontal disease and the patient's overall health. It is becoming more and more common for physicians to request specific dental information, i.e., perio exam and full mouth series (FMS), for reasons before unheard of. For example, I now have physicians requesting both for patients with serious abnormal EKG results. Patients needing knee replacement surgery or pacemaker placements are viewed by their physicians as needing complete periodontal workups prior to any surgery. This is simply further evidence that the dental patient is far more therapeutically complex than simply the oral cavity.

The now-well-established link between periodontal disease and many other systemic disorders is precisely why case treatment acceptance is fundamentally easier to obtain today than in the 1980s or before. This is an aggressive, oral-debilitating disease which produces endotoxins that in turn, inundate the tissues. These toxins proceed to perforate the tissue attachment which protects the bone. This allows for the destruction of the tooth's supporting structures. This by itself is bad enough, but there's more—a lot more.

Periodontal disease has been linked to heart disease, stroke, diabetes, premature births, Alzheimer's disease, dementia, arthritis, and even cancer. It lowers the body's immunity, making the body much more susceptible to contracting *any* disease, not the least of which is cancer. By the simple acts of chewing, eating or brushing one's teeth, oral bacteria find access to the bloodstream, move to all parts of the circulatory system, attract platelets, and with the influences of inflammation, cause clotting, which can lead to heart attacks and strokes.

- Eighty-five million Americans have some form of heart disease, while 200 million Americans have some form of gum disease. Patients with periodontal disease are twice as likely to have heart disease, which may be a higher cardiac risk than those with high cholesterol. *Streptococcus sanguinis*, a periopathogenic bacteria, has been linked to narrowed arteries, reduced blood flow, and ultimately, strokes. Every forty seconds, someone has a stroke in the United States. Every four minutes, someone dies of a stroke in the United States. I truly believe dentists and dental team members can contribute to the reduction in strokes and cardiovascular disease by simply addressing this problem via the treatment of periodontal disease, thereby reducing the volume of periopathogenic bacteria in the bloodstream.

- Diabetes and periodontal disease work both ways. If you are diabetic, you tend to develop periodontal disease, and if you have periodontal disease, you tend to develop diabetes.

- Pregnancy also presents complications for those women presenting with periodontal disease. Fifty to 70 percent of all women will develop some form of gum disease during pregnancy. Certain oral bacteria associated with periodontal disease, P. gingivalis and C. rectus, raise the risk of preterm birth if present during pregnancy. The American Academy of Periodontology (AAP) issued a position statement in 2004 stating that the treatment of periodontal disease in pregnant women is safe in the second trimester, and studies have shown reduced preterm birth rates among women treated during pregnancy versus those who delayed treatment until postpartum.

- Alzheimer's disease and dementia have also shown links to periodontal disease. Six periopathogenic spirochetes have been isolated in the brains of Alzheimer's patients, and there is a significant association between these spirochetes and the presence of Alzheimer's disease.

- Arthritis and periodontal disease show a commonality of pathogenesis. Both are forms of chronic inflammation, both exist in a soft tissue site, and both are adjacent to bone. They also show the release of the same inflammatory mediators (IL-1, IL-6, TNF-A1PHA, etc.).

- Cancer risks in studies have also shown to increase in the presence of periodontal disease. Periodontal disease bacteria produce toxins which weaken the immune system and cause the release of C-reactive proteins. This leads to inflamed blood vessels, which make it easier for bacteria (toxins) to attach to vascular linings, leading to the increased risk of cancer (lung, kidney, and blood cancers), all in the presence of periodontal disease.

All of these risks and complications occur because gum disease happens to be the body's most abundant source of low-grade inflammation. This omnipresent source of systemic inflammation tends to reduce the immune response and cause irreversible damage to the immune system.

The ultimate conclusion to all of this evidence is that we, as dental practitioners, dentists and hygienists, should know we are no longer simply treating the mouth, but instead the entire body.

## Treating The Periodontal Infection Cascade

The mouth is a wonderful place if you have infection, because it has a great blood supply and heals in spite of what we do to it. The mouth is also a terrible place if you have infection, because it has a great blood supply and will pick up that infection and circulate it throughout the body's bloodstream, influencing every other piece of tissue and body organ to some extent. This bombardment, twenty-four hours a day, seven days a week, 365 days a year, inevitably will force something to give way after a period of twenty, forty or sixty years.

The best way to look at periodontal disease is as a pyramid of infection. The base of the pyramid consists of the least-aggressive bacteria, and as you climb toward the apex of the pyramid, the bacteria increase in severity. Each group of bacteria build the base for the colonization of the next, more aggressive group. The most damaging bacteria sit at the apex of this pyramid.

The sole purpose of scaling and root planning is to destroy as much of this pyramid as possible. The physical removal via magnetostrictive or piezo devices is the only way to tear down this pyramid; it cannot be accomplished via rinse or pills. Once demolished, both antibiotics and high concentrations of oxygen can be used as needed to suppress the rise of the bacterial population. Antibiotics are of use, but not for prolonged purposes as the bacteria can develop resistance to the antibiotic. The use of high concentrated levels of oxygen, on the other hand, can be used for the sustained control of periodontal disease (see the company known as PerioProtect) in which the use of oxygen in a 1.7% prescription gel of hydrogen peroxide is carried via prescription trays to all needed sites intra-orally. Oracare (a rinse) is also very effective in the biofilm breakdown, is antiviral, and destroys volatile sulfuric compounds that cause bad breath. These are both highly effective products for the control of periodontal disease, replacing the dependency upon antibiotics.

Systemic antibiotic prescriptions may also have the drawback of not being filled by the patient or not being taken as directed. They also tend to unnecessarily affect the entire body, which in most cases is overkill. If the antibiotic were delivered locally, the concentration at a given site would be much higher and little or no influence on the rest of the body occurs. However periodontal disease exists as a biofilm, which tends to be refractory to antibiotics and thus more difficult to control with the constant use of antibiotics.

# 9

# Dental Hygiene Department Insanity

You've probably heard the popular expression that the definition of insanity is doing the same thing over and over again but expecting a different result. Most dental hygiene departments can relate to that definition—they see patients, clean their teeth, and send them home for six months. When patients return, their disease looks as bad or worse than it did before. And then, what do they do next? Why, they clean their teeth and send them home for six months. If there is *any* chance for a better result, then the system must change. The flaw here is always in the lack of a system: The fact that a structured periodontal system does not exist in the practice.

The five goals of periodontal therapy are:

- Eliminate subgingival pathogens

- Terminate the inflammatory process

- Enhance the attachment position

- Decrease pocket depths

- Keep the patient involved in the process

That final point is important. Once the patient's involvement in his or her own treatment ceases, then you have lost your periodontal program.

Periodontal disease operates through four stages: the bacteria first populate the root surface. Left there for sufficient time, they will begin to perforate the tissue attachment (the shield protecting the bone), and ultimately will destroy the plate of bone. Lastly, the healing phase begins.

Periodontal disease can be identified by way of five indicators:

1. Identify the bacteria.

2. Measure the bone loss.

3. With the use of the periodontal probe, document sites of attachment loss.

4. Record bleeding points (potentially 168, if twenty-eight teeth are present).

5. Last but not least, document evidence of any suppuration, exudate, or, as we call it in Chenoa, "*puuussss.*"

I have always instructed my hygienists to verbalize this way, because "*puuussss*" sounds disgusting. Am I trying to "gross the patient out?" *Absolutely*! I've gone as far as looking at the patient and saying, "If you had an abscess on your hand, would you suck it? Well, what do you think is happening here?" Patients are swallowing this exudate twenty-four hours a day, seven days a week, 365 days a year. And, it's feeding the bloodstream the same way. Sometimes you have to be graphic with your patients, and personally, I love to be graphic. In fact, *I can't get enough of it.* I have also educated my patients that periodontal disease operates exactly the same as cancer, inasmuch as it goes through periods of remission and exacerbation. In the early years of presenting this information, I told patients that periodontal disease "won't kill you," but it could take the life of the tooth. Due to the link between periodontal disease and systemic disorders, I no longer say this; rather, I now say that periodontal disease will not only take the life of your tooth, or teeth, but may also contribute to your own shortened life expectancy.

Smoking is an amazing contributor to the existence of periodontal disease, by the way it leads to chronic inflammation. Whether they are past or present smokers, smoking contributes to 53 percent of all gum disease associated with adult dental patients. Simply asking if your patients are current or past smokers will give you a very good idea of the prevalence of periodontal disease in your existing patient base, even before you place a probe in the patient's mouth.

## The D-Word

One word used too infrequently in our profession by both dentists and hygienists is the word "disease." Every night before going to sleep, all dentists and hygienists need to look in the mirror and say *disease* three times, then go to sleep, get up the next day, go to the office, look at the first patient in hygiene, and say, "How does it feel to know that you are a periodontally diseased human being?" Watch their eyes open to the size of silver dollars; they know what that word means and they do *not* want to own it.

Next, the patient will likely ask, "Am I going to lose my teeth? Can you save my teeth? Am I going to need dentures?" The moment any one of those questions arises, the patient has already accepted your periodontal program—*and you haven't even quoted the cost*. Patients won't ask the questions unless they want to fix the problem, and they *all* ask.

Periodontal disease is a symptomless disease. Therefore it is imperative that all staff members develop appropriate education, communication, and listening skills. The disease and its treatment permeate all aspects of the dental practice. This is illustrated by the fact that proper words and phrases must be utilized. Instead of *gum inflammation, scaling, root planning*, and *bleeding*, words or phrases such as *disease, infection, hemorrhaging* and *periodontal therapy* are far more suitable and effective. Continually emphasize that periodontal disease can *only* be controlled; it cannot be cured. The patient must value the service and their participation is not only essential but vital to their success and management of this disease.

In non-surgical periodontal therapy, I advocate the treatment of three case types: I, II and III.

- Case Type I utilizes the code D4346 and requires the presence of suprabony pockets and generalized bleeding. Treatment is generally accomplished via a single one-hour therapy appointment followed by a thirty-minute re-evaluation visit, usually one week post-op. Keep Case Type I patients on a three-month maintenance schedule, because short of that, the inflammation invariably returns and treatment must be repeated. Maintenance, like oil changes, keeps the cost at manageable levels for the patient. In 2018, the fee range for Case Type I patients is approximately $500–$650.

- Case Type II patients represent 80 percent of all case types treated in the dental practice. These patients are generally associated with actual bone loss (not simply suprabony pockets). Pocket depth range here is three to five millimeters, and the code utilized to treat these patients is D4341. Case Type II patients are generally treated by side of the mouth (left or right), both upper and lower arches on a given side, and in a timeframe of one hour per side of the mouth. The thirty-minute re-evaluation is done approximately one week post-op. The current fee range for Case Type II patients is approximately $1,150–$1550.

- Case Type III patients are treated by quadrants, one hour per quadrant, but this periodontal disease therapy is a flexible system. For example, if the hygienist requests two hours for the LR quadrant and one hour each for the other three quadrants, then that is exactly the amount of time he or she should receive for treatment. There may be mitigating circumstances, such as more teeth, deeper pockets, more subgingival calculus, or even furcation involvement. The fee is based on how much time is spent to treat that particular patient and case type. Case Type III patients generally present with four- to six-millimeter pockets. All therapy is treated under the code D4341 for the instrumentation of the crown and root and is not prophylactic in nature, followed by a one-week post-op re-evaluation visit (thirty minutes). D4342 is a code to be used for smaller, isolated numbers of teeth, groups of generally one to three teeth, and is also a therapeutic, not prophylactic, code. The only criteria required to use D4341 or D4342 is the presence of disease. The fee range for a Case Type III periodontal patient is currently $1,600–$2,200.

## The Price Of Oral-Systemic Health

All dental practices, one way or another, face the issue of collecting out-of-pocket payments from their patients. The fact that perio-educated patients know that this disease is not only harmful to their teeth but also their overall health, and that it is not curable but must be constantly monitored, makes out-of-pocket collection much easier to navigate.

Most insurance companies pay for prophys twice per year, and if additional visits are needed, then the patient assumes responsibility. The problem is that the dentists feel as though their patients will pay nothing out of pocket. Fortunately, that isn't true. The periodontally-educated patient knows that perio maintenance visits are synonymous with an oil change for their car or truck, whereas periodontal therapy is a new transmission with respect to cost. If they don't elect to pay for a few oil changes (inexpensive), then they will ultimately have to pay for the transmission (periodontal therapy). They understand if they choose not to pay for periodontal therapy, then they will at some point be forced to pay for extractions, partials, dentures, and ultimately, a potentially shortened life expectancy. Untreated periodontal disease leads to fewer teeth and more inefficient chewing (about 300+ psi for your own teeth versus about 50 psi with a set of dentures); improperly and inefficiently chewed food leads to poor digestion of that food, poor nutrient absorption of undigested food, and thus, further systemic disorders and, obviously, a shortened life expectancy. As you can see, this is a downward spiral if left untreated. Eating, digesting, and absorbing nutrients are essential to a long and healthy life.

# 10

# Dental Plan Confidential
## Dental insurance is *not* insurance.

That statement alone should raise some eyebrows. If it doesn't, you're probably comatose. This is, in my opinion, where dentists have chosen to lose their identity, because dentists tend to hold dental insurance as the Holy Grail of their profession. Dental insurance seems to dictate every decision made in a dental practice, for better or worse, and it's mostly for worse! As a profession, we view dental insurance as the barometer regarding whether a patient can afford treatment or not.

It goes without saying that we tend to treatment-plan the insurance— not the patient. A patient without dental insurance is looked upon as someone who "can't afford anything," simply because they lack insurance. I view this in exactly the opposite fashion. Meaning, I see the patient without insurance as the *best* opportunity for case treatment acceptance, and here's why: The uninsured patient has not been limited regarding what they will spend by way of an artificial insurance budget. The insurance industry, consciously or not, educates our patients that if the insurance company does not cover a procedure, or does not pay entirely for a procedure, then the procedure is not a true dental "necessity." If the procedure is necessary, then their policy will cover it, and *cover* means every dime.

In other words, if insurance doesn't pay every nickel for a crown, then the crown is *obviously not necessary.*

Patients without dental insurance have no such preconceived ideas or restrictions. I have spent years in my practice educating patients not to renew dental insurance as part of their next employment contract. I implore them to research the dollars taken out of their check each day to pay for a dental policy and, as I previously mentioned in Chapter 2, invest this money to pay for their own dentistry. Why continue to pay for benefits they don't use and that pay so little towards their overall dental care?

Insurance is protection against the occurrence of an infrequent, catastrophic event. Dentistry, on the other hand, involves the frequent occurrence of noncatastrophic events. Hence, as previously stated, dental insurance is *not*, by definition, insurance. Dental insurance is rather a benefit to help defray the costs of quality care, or even simply a form of health care financing. But it's not "coverage," as this word implies "complete," and there is nothing complete about dental insurance. The dental insurance plan is nothing more than a contract between the employer and the designated insurance company—not the patient. The patient has little control over the purchased policy, as it is generally one that the employer can afford, regardless of whether or not it is the best policy for that given employee. To the best of my knowledge, there are no dental insurance plans that are all-inclusive of what a patient may need or desire during a lifetime for optimal dental care. It is therefore imperative to educate patients that they must supplement their dental insurance benefits, particularly during the lifetime of a non-curable disease such as periodontal disease.

I have more than a few egregious issues within my own profession, but one of the biggest is the idea of feeling obligated to participate in dental insurance plans. Once a dentist commits to going down this road, your talents, abilities and knowledge as a practicing dentist cease to be relevant. At this point, the dentist can no longer provide what patients need or desire, but instead, only what your membership in the plan entitles you to offer. The plan now dictates your every spoken word and the range of services that can be offered to that patient. These "participating member" plans are so restrictive upon the dentists that they are told what they can do, when they can do it, and how much they are going to be paid for it. *Please tell me the difference between that and the oldest profession in the world.*

The plan dictates your every move, not the needs of the patient. When a patient presents with obvious needs, the fact that you, as a dentist, already know the restrictions put upon you by that policy may preempt you from presenting the appropriate treatment plan to the patient.

I could never practice dentistry with such a noose around my neck.

When I treatment-plan my patients, I refuse any prior knowledge of their insurance plans or coverage. I treatment-plan patients, not their insurance plans, and certainly not their wallets. Their finances are irrelevant to me; whether the patient has insurance or whether they can afford my proposal, I must still tell them the truth. It's not my job to evaluate my patients in regard to their financial status or their insurance coverage. I'm a dentist, not an investigator or a soothsayer.

The suffocating parameters placed on dentists who participate in these plans make it impossible to properly treatment-plan a patient, and I have expressed all of these thoughts to my patients in order for them to appreciate the fact that I will only tell them the truth—not what they (or their insurance company) want to hear. It's probably just me, but in no way could I sleep at night if those restraints were put on me each day while practicing my profession.

## You Have To Be Able To Sleep At Night

In the early 1990s I was offered an opportunity by a person who, at that time, I considered to be a close friend. He spoke with me about a life-changing, wealth-accumulating endeavor in dentistry that on its surface appeared intriguing and extremely tempting. About forty minutes into our discussion, I broached the question: "What is your overall objective or philosophy in all of this? What is your mission statement?"

His response was, "Well, Bob, what we do is prophylactic dentistry," which caused me to ask, "What the hell is that?" He then proceeded to explain to me that "prophylactic dentistry" means that if tooth number two required an occlusal restoration, then we also restore teeth three, four and five.

I responded, "But those additional teeth were not decayed."

He replied, "Well, if number two is decayed, then it's only a matter of time before teeth three, four, and five will also be decayed."

I said, "So, you are restoring teeth that are not decayed because you feel they eventually will be decayed, right?"

"Exactly."

I said, "This is where we go our separate ways." I told him that I have to be able to sleep at night, and if I practiced like that, there would be no chance of any peace. I've been told by acquaintances of his over the years that I lost millions of dollars by not taking that "opportunity." No; I made millions the right way, by telling people the truth and offering and providing the highest quality care I know to each patient. There are things far greater than money in life, and I believe you reap what you sow. So no, I didn't miss out on anything. Sorry to go biblical, but life is a blink of an eye, and eternity is forever. I always want to know I'm in my "right place," and I won't sell my soul for money or anything else.

# 11

## On Treatment, Reimbursement, Butt-In-Chair Time, and Guilt: *A Different Mindset*

Going back to the discussion of dental plans: I am a realist, and I know that being involved in such plans requires the doctor to work harder for far less reward. Dentists have strength in numbers, meaning these plans could not exist if dentists simply refused to play.

I am not talking collusion here, but a simple reassessment of your core values regarding why you became a dentist in the first place. One reason had to be self-employment (being your own boss). A second may have been a desire to work with your hands, but in a controlled environment. Last, but not least, was likely the desire to control your own destiny and your own financial future. Two of these three are out the door if you are a participating member of those dental plans (in network).

If enough (not all) dentists looked at themselves in the mirror and recommitted to these ideals, then it would be very difficult and unprofitable for insurance companies to operate the way they do. It is the fear of losing patients that drives dentists into these plans in the first place, and it is very simple to explain to patients that while participating in those plans, you, the doctor cannot even offer them all of the quality solutions to a problem, but only those authorized by the plan. On the contrary, not being a participating member allows you, as a doctor, to offer any treatment plan and allow the patient to choose their level of quality care ... not only that dictated by the plan.

I personally believe that periodontal disease is treated properly by such a small percentage of dentists (and evidence supports this), that they will inevitably lose the privilege of being able to treat it. Insurance companies have learned that when patients with certain chronic conditions receive care for their periodontal disease, the patients' health care costs drop significantly. The central theme of most dental practices, however, is delivering high-cost restorative care; treating periodontal disease isn't even an afterthought. This is a *huge mistake*, not only in terms of quality of care for our patients, but also in terms of economics. It is becoming more and more apparent that both insurers and employers are motivated to control health care costs. The fact that periodontal disease impacts many other previously mentioned systemic disorders makes it nearly inevitable that the treatment of this disease will get packaged into overall medical care. What should be obvious here is that insurance companies *want* this disease treated, whether the dentist wants to treat it or not. Quite simply, this means that physicians may inevitably sponsor the treatment of periodontal disease.

Again, if dentists don't want to treat periodontal disease (and most apparently don't), then it is only logical that such treatment be provided by the medical profession. This is, after all, a disease, right? Physicians treat disease, too. Just because it is an oral disease won't prevent treatment by the medical profession if pressure is sufficiently applied by the insurance industry. If it is apparent (and it is) that dentists aren't doing their part to control the systemic effects of this disease, then responsibility for managing and treating periodontal disease will be rightfully turned over to the medical profession.

I can't fathom why a dentist would *not* treat a disease that is the number one cause of tooth loss, affects a higher percentage of their patients than anything else, and receives greater acceptance by patients than anything else proposed in a dental practice. A periodontal treatment plan is accepted almost universally, if properly presented. There are patients who do not care if they save all of their teeth, but not one patient wants to contribute to their own shortened life expectancy. Anything proposed to a patient that forces them to observe their own mortality will be accepted sooner or later.

An insurance plan may not cover all procedures, or the entire cost of those procedures, but that should *not* prevent dentists from advising the patient of their needs, or even providing services, provided they are not submitted to an insurance company for reimbursement. Simply diagnose all of the patient's needs and give the patient the opportunity to pay for it. Insurance companies are not in business, nor should they be, to solve all of a patient's needs. Rather, they are in business to make money. Period.

Crown-and-bridge mindset versus periodontal mindset are markedly different in the eyes of a typical dentist. The doctor values crown and bridge, but does not value the periodontal aspects of his or her practice.

What does the average dentist charge for a crown procedure in 2018? About $1,000. How many times (technology aside) does that same dentist see the patient in order to complete the crown and its delivery? Two times.

As for the first appointment for that crown, I am not interested in how much time is on the schedule, but rather how much time the doctor's butt is in the chair: We shall call this "butt-in-chair time." Butt-in-chair time doesn't start until the doctor's butt touches the chair to provide the anesthetic. Once the procedure is completed, the clock stops. The clock doesn't restart until the doctor's butt hits the chair again in order to prepare the tooth. Once the impression tray is in the mouth, the clock again stops, and usually doesn't start again. So, what's the total butt-in-chair time for the first appointment for the crown? About twenty minutes. Clock it with a stopwatch and you will see it's very close.

Next is the second and final appointment for the crown. Here, the crown is delivered (cemented to place) and the butt-in-chair time here is about five minutes, assuming a quality lab with predictable results. However, let's say we've got a PITA (pain-in-the-a**—more about them later) and the time is ten minutes. After all this, you can easily see that the total butt-in-chair time was about thirty minutes, and how much did you charge for the crown? That's right: $1,000. Therefore, "butt in chair" time generated $2,000 per hour.

I'm sure the dentist feels no guilt or remorse, and the reasons for this are many: The crown is a work of art. It took years to create, and we just waited for someone to need it. The crown is also made of pure gold, mined in California three weeks ago, and most of all, there is a lab bill to cover. The lab bill was $999; the doctor made a mere dollar, and the patient knows this because we have subtle ways of getting the point across. Now, let me ask a question: How many teeth did you treat for $1,000? One, that's how many.

I'm asking and advocating that you instead treat twelve teeth, twenty teeth, thirty teeth for a comparable fee to the $1,000 *and stop feeling guilty about it*. What's more beneficial: Treating one tooth for that price, or removing the infection around twenty-eight such teeth for a similar price? If you want to feel guilty about something, then feel guilty about the fact that you charged $1,000 to put a crown on a tooth that was swimming in a cesspool of infection. *That* is something to feel guilty about.

# 12

# The Biggest Prophy Mistake

A prophy cannot be therapeutic and does not involve subgingival procedures. Knowing this, ask yourself, doctors: Are you providing therapeutic procedures and charging prophy fees? Of course you are. Don't feel bad. We all are, or have, and it's costing you hundreds of thousands of dollars per year to continue making this mistake.

Achieving case treatment acceptance of periodontal therapy programs should involve the doctor as little as possible. Dentists frequently feel an obligation to enter the hygiene treatment room and put their two cents into the presentation. If that were all the doctor contributed, it would be great, but it isn't. Instead of two cents, they put in a buck-and-a-half, and consequently talk the patient out of the case treatment acceptance (ironically, prior to their entering the room, the hygienist had already accomplished it). The doctor may say something like, "Well, Mrs. Smith, this is definitely something we need to put a watch on." (Seriously? If you want to watch something, doctor, then rent a movie. Periodontal disease does not go away by "watching it." It only gets worse.)

Gaining case treatment acceptance and keeping the patient involved in the process require that every employee in the practice feels comfortable answering any and all questions about perio therapy. This requirement does not apply only to the doctor and the hygienist. In fact, the person asked most of the questions will be sitting at the front desk. Patients feel that front desk staff members are not as qualified to answer these questions; and in fact, patients are banking on it.

If a patient approaches the front desk and asks, "What's this periodontal stuff all about?" and the response is, "I'm not sure, maybe you should go back there and ask them—I don't get back there very often," the patient's first thought now is, "You work here and don't know why this is being treated. Why should I worry about treating it?" A staff member has effectively just given the patient the justification for not treating their periodontal disease, which is exactly what the patient was looking for.

Doctors have their own fears about initiating a periodontal therapy program. The dreaded fear associated with the question, "Why haven't we done this *before*?" coming from existing patients will literally send them running for the tall grass. And yet, the question is easy to answer if you know how.

Simply explain to the patient that your office has been attempting to control this invasive disease for years, but most patients are taking two steps forward and three steps back, and this losing ground is resulting in losing bone, which supports the patient's teeth. Thus, you have been highly focused in your continuing education, taking courses to not only learn more about this disease and how it operates, but also to learn how to properly treat this disease. And today, dentists have a state-of-the-art system which is providing positive results for patients. We are now able to arrest the disease and place all of our patients on a customized maintenance program to continue its control, because the disease itself cannot be cured. The key is that by controlling this disease, we can limit further damage and limit its negative contributions to the patient's overall health. This is the point at which you emphasize (or re-emphasize) links between periodontal disease and specific systemic disorders, noting those associated with that patient. It is now appropriate to say, "I'm sure this is something you would like to get under control, Mrs. Smith. How soon can we get your therapy started?"

All patients are probed six points per tooth at every hygiene visit, with the exception of any therapy appointments. The probe readings dictate everything. For example, if the patient has completed their periodontal therapy, are in maintenance, and all indicators are good, all numbers are three or less, no bleeding, no subgingival calculus, no furcation involvements, and no exudate, then no therapy is required and the patient is in line for a prophylaxis. If, however, all these qualifiers are *not* met, then a periodontal treatment plan is developed based on the collected information. The time allotted to develop this plan should be between four to six minutes. Here the patient is case typed, assigned a fee, and presented their customized treatment plan. The patient can now either be kept to fill any downtime in the hygiene schedule or re-appointed for a subsequent visit.

Fees are always based on time required to provide the therapy, as time is money. Two hours of therapy should not cost the same as one hour of therapy. This has always seemed common sense to me. Every procedure I have ever performed has been timed with a stopwatch— not to see how fast I can perform it, but to see how long it takes me to perform the procedure the right way. In this way, I place a dollar amount on what I feel I am worth per hour to provide dentistry. All procedures that I perform are charged out at a percentage of what that dollar amount happens to be, depending upon the length of time required to complete the given procedure.

Once patients have completed the periodontal therapy program, they are placed in a customized maintenance program and seen every ninety days. As touched on previously, a prophy and a periodontal maintenance visit are not the same; a prophy cannot control disease, but periodontal maintenance is designed to do just that. Prophies are supragingival and play no role in the control of this disease. *Periodontal maintenance and prophies are not synonymous.* Periodontal maintenance debrides the sulcular sites of both attached and nonattached bacteria. A prophy doesn't even go there. A subgingival disease (periodontal) cannot be controlled by supragingival plaque control (prophy).

A great way to express this to your patients is, "We can't get rid of a problem above the gumline in order to treat a disease located below the gumline." Makes perfect sense, doesn't it? If you are going to provide periodontal therapy, then you must provide periodontal maintenance or be considered negligent. Once a patient agrees to begin periodontal therapy, it is imperative to inform the patient that periodontal maintenance is required every ninety days and explain why.

# 13

# Periodontal Disease Is a Monster Problem

Periodontal disease is unique and bizarre in how it operates, as it appears to jump around the oral cavity for no apparent reason. But there *are* reasons. Systemic contributions, lack of oral hygiene, stress, and the inability to maintain proper maintenance schedules all are reasons for this malady. This explains why, from one visit to the next, the mouth can exhibit apparently healthy tissue or can show flare-ups of bleeding and pocketing.

In 1981, Dr. Jefferson Hardin, a periodontist, wrote in the *Journal of Public Health Dentistry* about the worldwide prevalence of periodontal disease, and that its occurrence was apparent from the first decade of life through old age. Dr. Hardin was clearly ahead of his time when he alluded to the fact that general dentists' involvement in the control of this disease was not only necessary but imperative if there were any chance to control it. There are not enough periodontists to even get a handle on this disease, and those same periodontists do not want their chairs occupied with scaling and root planning patients; they want to see surgery and implant patients.

It is difficult for me to imagine why a general dentist would have to be forced to do something (and it's coming to that) that is of such benefit to both the patient and the general practice. Treating periodontal disease dramatically enhances the quality of care for the patient while limiting the doctor's liability. In the process, the patient's life expectancy can potentially be extended while allowing the doctor to win the dentistry lottery.

One of the largest pitfalls in the successful implementation of a periodontal therapy program is the habitual use of the word "cleaning." It is imperative to remove this word from your dental vocabulary. The only appropriate use of the word "cleaning" is if the phone rings and the prospective patient says, "I want to make an appointment for a cleaning." The appropriate response here is, "We offer two types of cleanings in our office: One for patients that have healthy gums, bone, and teeth, and one for those who don't. We do not know which category you fall into until we do an exam."

Now, 99 percent of patients will respond, "Sure, sounds good. I will see you Tuesday at 8:00 a.m." The only other possible response would be, "Well, I don't want an exam." In thirty years of providing periodontal therapy, only one patient has responded in that manner. He came into my office wanting a new upper partial denture. Upon seating him, my hygienist stated that we would be needing to collect some information via a couple of exams prior to discussing the new upper partial. He was informed that our first exam was designed to evaluate the bone support that was needed for his new partial. The patient made it clear he wasn't interested in any exams; he just wanted his new upper partial. When I was informed of this, I entered the hygiene treatment room and explained that the periodontal exam would determine if the upper partial was even an option for him. Well, long story short, the patient refused the periodontal exam and I referred him to a periodontist, which he quickly declined. So, no partial.

I didn't *lose* the partial; I *did* avoid a potential lawsuit. Because if a new partial were to have "rocked" his teeth loose within any period of time, that patient likely would have been the first person to sue me for negligence.

If a patient presents with generalized bleeding on probing, subgingival calculus, and pocketing, and receives a "cleaning," then that patient is leaving the dentist's office with active infection, which represents malpractice on the part of the dentist. And that applies whether the patient wanted a new partial or not.

## Time Is Money—And Oral Health

A well-known statistic in our profession is that 3 percent of hygienists' production is from the use of the 4000 codes—those codes used to treat periodontal disease. It is also known that the level of periodontal services compared to overall hygiene production *is less than 1 percent*. These two facts are another way of saying that periodontal services essentially do not even exist in the vast majority of dental practices. This is further reinforced by simply asking a dental practice about their hygiene periodontal program. The two most common responses are, "What program?" and "Yeah, we're getting started on that." In both cases, that means *it doesn't exist*.

In regard to periodontal maintenance visits, the question is always, "How much time do you block for such a visit?" Since 1988, with the structured periodontal system in place, I have blocked thirty minutes for all periodontal maintenance appointments. Now, before the dentists or hygienists reading this go into a state of shock, please understand the only requirement during the thirty-minute visit is to probe the patient. This is a procedure that normally requires five to six minutes of the hygienist's time. Once probed, if the patient shows pink stippled tissue with no pocketing, no bleeding, and no other indication of active disease, a prophy is in order. If, however, bleeding, pocketing, and subgingival calculus are present, then the patient is case-typed and earmarked with the appropriate fee. The specific periodontal program is then presented to the patient. Upon acceptance (typically, again, more than 90 percent) and collection of out-of-pocket costs, the patient is kept to back-fill any down time on the schedule at $200–$400 per hour, or re-appointed for treatment at a subsequent visit.

I never thought I would say this, but in my first few years treating periodontal disease, I used to pray for hygiene cancellations (unimaginable, but true). The reason is any or all cancellations allowed me the opportunity to substitute quality care, periodontal therapy, at $200–$400 per hour for the now-cancelled bloody prophy. There is absolutely no service provided in dentistry that trumps periodontal therapy with respect to quality of care and financial benefits.

Periodontal disease affects everything we do in dentistry: implants, crown and bridge, cosmetic dentistry, even orthodontics, because teeth do not move predictably in the presence of inflammation.

Further evidence of the scarcity of periodontal therapy in the general dental practice lies in analytics that show 70 percent of all adult dental records do not contain full periodontal charting. Adding salt to the wound, 80 percent of the practice's patients have a disease that we are not treating by 20:1—the ratio by which prophys outnumber periodontal procedures. For the small percentage of patients who are actually treated for this disease, a majority (68 percent) are only seen zero to two times per year for periodontal maintenance visits. This, even though four maintenance visits per year are recommended. Knowing statistics like these, should anyone be surprised that 75 to 90 percent of American adults have periodontal disease?

If you observe your daily hygiene software printout, you will likely find that by a large margin, most of your codes are the 1110s. Also, observe the percentage of patient bibs that are bloody upon completion of your prophys, and you will see it is the vast majority. Most hygienists probably do the best they can with each patient, based on the time allotted by the doctor on the schedule, but they consistently have insufficient time to treat their patients. The reason for this is that the hygiene schedule is not designed to treat disease, as it is impossible to treat a disease in a thirty-, forty-, or sixty-minute window. The hygienist is providing his or her best scaling and root-planing abilities during this time, sending the patient to the front desk, and charging for a prophy. All of those scaling and root planning skills were given away, and yet the patient was not helped, as the task at hand was never completed. In essence, the tuxedo was placed on the proverbial garbage can. The garbage, periodontal disease, is still in the can; you just made it look cosmetically better.

The average national daily hygiene production in 2018 is about $1,100 per day. Eighty percent of periodontal therapy is represented by Case Type II patients. The average fee for these patients is about $1,350. It is therefore easy to see how one periodontal program per day will more than double that day's hygiene production, and it is virtually impossible (if properly presented) to receive acceptance of *only* one such case type per day in a dental office. Whereas most practices bill an average of 80 to 90 percent prophy codes (1110) per year, they should be billing 80 to 90 percent periodontal service codes (4000s). If only 10 percent of the billed codes were in the 4000s, the financial status of that practice would be unrecognizable.

Dentists commonly ask me, "Do I need a hygienist to initiate a periodontal program?" The answer is, "No, you don't." However, without a hygienist, you will have two to three weeks to hire one. Consider: if only two patients per day need and accept periodontal therapy (ludicrous, but let's go with it), and the average time to treat that patient, start to finish, is three hours, then at the end of the day, you will have booked six hours of periodontal therapy. By week's end, there would be twenty-four hours of periodontal therapy on the books. By the end of three weeks, there will be seventy-two hours of periodontal therapy on the books. Who is going to perform all of this treatment? The doctor? Well, if the doctor is involved in seventy-two hours of periodontal therapy, then who will do the restorative, dentures, partials, and endo? *Nobody, that's who.* The ideal scenario, therefore, is to delegate perio therapy to the hygiene department and *leave them alone.* The hygienists will run the system better than the doctor can in his or her wildest dreams. And for the first time in their lives as hygienists, they are no longer the cleaning people, but a highly productive part of your dental practice.

# 14

# Practice Management Considerations In Perio Therapy

C ancellations and no-shows in hygiene have been a thorn in the side of every dental practice. The solution to this problem came to me in late 1987, when I realized that every day, I had patients needing and accepting periodontal therapy, and I had two options for each of these patients: One, keep the patient and backfill the schedule at $200–$400 per hour, providing periodontal therapy; two, reappoint the patient and provide therapy at a subsequent dental visit.

For example, let's say a patient enters the office at 8:00 a.m., sits in the hygiene chair, and by 8:30 a.m., it's been established the patient has gingivitis. At 8:35 a.m., the phone rings, and it's Betty, the 9:00 a.m. patient. She cancels. Betty just gave you twenty-five minutes' notice. You might as well enjoy it, because it's twenty-five more minutes than you usually get.

Now, when this occurs, what does the doctor do? Does the doctor just disappear? No; the doctor enters his or her private office and remains there for about five minutes, then comes to the front desk, leans over the counter, looks down at the poor receptionist, and says, "How, ah … how's it going?"

Now the doctor turns away and retreats back into the private office— for about five more minutes. Then it's another trip to the front desk, looking down at the poor receptionist: "You, ah, you got anybody yet?" And while the doctor may not know it, it's highly likely that this question will be followed by a rather unpleasant hand gesture as he or she retreats to the private office again.

The problem here is you are asking the receptionist to call people, get them out of bed, shower, shave, dress them, and get them into the dental office in twenty-five minutes. That isn't going to happen. The best you could hope for is to salvage thirty of the next sixty minutes on the schedule. In most cases, you simply have to eat the entire sixty minutes. But what if the prospective next patient, who has gingivitis, is already sitting in the chair? *Now* what can you do? Well, you can give that patient *many* reasons to stay. If disease is treated at this level, it is the least extensive and the least expensive form to treat. If it is treated at this level, the patient can save the cost of gasoline to return later. Treated at this level, it requires *no needles*. A designated office person can now sit chairside and discuss the cost and out-of-pocket expense, which is the *least* you collect from that patient.

You have now successfully filled the 9:00 a.m.–10:00 a.m. void in your schedule, and at $200–$400 per hour (versus the $80–$100 which the original patient, Betty, was going to pay). Ninety-nine percent of the time, when you backfill the schedule with periodontal therapy, it will double or triple the production of the previously scheduled patient. As I'm sure is readily apparent, this system fills a logical need in any dental practice.

## No, Patients Really Are Not Flossing

One of my pet peeves in dentistry is that, for some strange reason, dental professionals *actually believe* many of their patients floss daily. Statistically, 5 percent of a patient population will floss consistently and effectively on a daily basis and to believe otherwise is ludicrous. Consider: 75 to 90 percent of the adult population has one form or another of periodontal disease. Assuming this is true (and it is), then how is it possible for many or most to be regular flossers? *It isn't.* You can't have it both ways.

The primary uses of dental floss in society are very likely skipping rope, tying shoes, holding ponytails, stitching wounds, and of course, the classic: weaving a rope to escape prison. (This actually occurred in 1994, when an inmate used forty-eight strands of mint-flavored waxed floss, braided to the thickness of a telephone cord, in order to escape from a recreational yard in prison.) The point is that floss is being used for many things, but the epidemiological evidence suggests that placing it interproximally and subgingivally to help prevent a disease is not high on the list.

## Don't Leave Revenue On The Table (Or Patients Untreated In The Chair)

There is no debating that periodontal disease is obvious and prevalent in *all* dental practices. The disease doesn't care where you live, how much money you have, or even how well educated you are. It happens to be so rampant in American society that 80 percent of adults have mild to moderate periodontal disease. Once you reach the age of fifty-five and older, that number jumps to 90 percent, most of whom are categorized as moderate to severe periodontal patients.

The fact that this insidious disease cannot be cured means it must be monitored, controlled, and treated throughout the lifetime of the patient. Imagine four to six patients per day needing and accepting periodontal therapy at fees ranging from $1,100–$2,000. That, doctor, is the same scenario as having four to six patients per day accepting crown-and-bridge therapy. And you, the doctor, do not have to personally treat it; you can delegate treatment to your hygiene department. Delegation of duties becomes even more appreciated the older the doctor becomes, because at some point, you'll have to cut back on your production. And on the other side of the practice, the beautiful thing about this system for the hygienist is that he or she will never again be limited in the time allotted to treat a patient; instead, the hygienist tells the doctor how much time is needed to properly treat the patient. And regardless of whether two hours or eight hours are needed, the fee is always based on the amount of time required to treat that patient. This customization is exactly why this system so successfully treats this disease.

When patients are diagnosed medically for deep wounds, stomach ulcers, broken bones, or debilitating diseases, each case is not treated the same, nor with identical techniques. In the same way, the cost is not the same, depending on the circumstances. It should be no different in dentistry; all patients are different, and they all present their own unique challenges. That is why the treatment plans and costs should vary accordingly.

A majority of dentists in 2018 say that they are not busy enough. This is a problem that has been trending since the early 1970s. So, in review, dentists are not as busy as they would like to be; 75 to 90 percent of the adult population has periodontal disease; and the level of periodontal services rendered by general dentists is less than 1 percent.

Can anyone see a logical fit here? This, combined with the fact that more than 90 percent of insurance claims are not for periodontal services, leads to a stark conclusion: 80 percent of our patients have a disease that represents less than 10 percent of the insurance claims.

## Time To Ditch The PSR?

The Periodontal Screening and Recording (PSR) has been used improperly for decades in our profession. It is only a screening tool; it should not and cannot be used for diagnostic purposes in a dental setting. In my opinion, the only useful purpose of a PSR in dentistry is for an emergency patient. For example, a patient enters the office needing or wanting an extraction. After seating the patient and reviewing the medical history, it is observed that the patient does have one or more systemic disorder(s) that are easily linked to the effects of periodontal disease. The next step is to provide the anesthesia for the extraction. Once complete, it is now time to provide the PSR (thirty seconds) and simply determine if periodontal disease does in fact exist or not (no case typing, no treatment plan, no fees) by spot-probing the mouth. Now, extract the tooth. While the patient is resting comfortably post-extraction, begin educating that patient about the link between periodontal disease and their systemic disorders.

This process, post-extraction, generally requires six to ten minutes. This is routinely done in my practice; in more than 90 percent of all cases, the patient will pay for the extraction and then appoint for their initial periodontal exam. This leads to a very high rate of acceptance of periodontal therapy and subsequent restorative treatment, as periodontal education drives restorative treatment.

## When Compassion Is Dangerous

Hygienists, as a rule, tend to underdiagnose to save patients money or provide the periodontal therapy at no charge to the patient. I understand compassion and the urge not to diagnose periodontal disease for the sake of saving the patient money. But by doing so, they are not doing the patient any favors. On the contrary, by ignoring the disease hygienists are putting patients' overall systemic health at risk. The other, more frequent problem (previously noted) is that the hygienists are scaling and root planning during prophy visits and are not charging for it. This *also* isn't helping the patient or the practice, but is of great benefit to the bottom line of the insurance company. The hygienist gets into this predicament, doing both the scaling and prophy in the same visit, because they are not scheduled to allow for therapy—only a prophy. The problem now arises when that same patient is referred to a specialist or transfers to another office. At that point, if the periodontal condition has not been documented or billed, then your office is liable.

In order for a hygienist to provide quality periodontal therapy, the system must be in place, the technology to provide that therapy must be available, they must be supported by the doctor and the team, and (of course) financial rewards should be provided for all team members involved. I will focus on an example of these rewards later, but suffice it to say all team members should be rewarded based entirely upon their contribution to the system. Since periodontal disease is essentially symptomless, the value of having a system in place is imperative. The information must be collected properly, all patient questions answered in a timely and complete fashion, and the right presentation (there are many wrong ones) must be made to the patient. These steps lead to near-universal acceptance by the patient, which sets the patient up for the appropriate periodontal therapy program and a customized maintenance schedule.

I have heard about twenty-five to thirty questions over a thirty-year period treating this disease, and I have created a dialogue pack which includes these questions and how to properly answer them. Role-playing and rehearsal using this packet will provide doctor and staff with all the cover you need in your presentation. (See dialogue pack in appendix C.)

Unfortunately, dentists today still tend to believe that the way to enhance production is by working more hours and seeing more patients. Sadly, that is merely the way to end up with one foot in the grave and the other on a banana peel. Hygiene production is not driven upward by seeing a higher volume of patients or by working longer hours. Counterintuitively, it is driven upward by reducing the volume of patients and dramatically raising the quality of care. Work smarter, not harder; when you are working longer hours, seeing more patients, then your stress levels go up, salaries increase, supply usage elevates, and you use more utilities. A single hygiene treatment room with a structured periodontal program can see three to four patients per day and generate three to five times the income of a nonperiodontal day, seeing eight patients in the same amount of time. Periodontal therapy allows you to raise the quality of care for all patients in your practice, working far less, and generating substantially more money.

# 15

# Is It All Worth It? Factoring In The PITA Factor And More

The PITA (pain in the a**) factor: We've all got patients who have it, and they take time off of our body clocks. Do you know what that means? It means they are going to kill you!

These patients traumatized me for years in private practice and I felt obligated to treat them. No, I didn't want to treat them, but I had to, for the same reason you have to. *I needed the income*! But once periodontal therapy was launched in my practice, there was no more obligation to treat all of these stressful scenarios. They were now routinely referred, to allow someone else who specialized in treating that kind of stress to deal with it. The PITAs were now routinely plucked from my schedule, and I was left with a far more productive and far less stressful day. I could once again begin to look at the next day's schedule and felt no further obligation to provide services I did not enjoy. The well-documented stress in dentistry was always the reason I liked, but didn't love, my job.

Periodontal therapy allowed all of that to change. I no longer felt the burden to heal all wounds, as I was now able to allow someone else to do that which I didn't want to do, or was not as qualified to do.

## From Nightmare to Dream Patient With Perio Therapy

In early 1988, a patient entered my practice for a new exam. And after seating him, my hygienist walked up to me and said, "You might as well forget about this one."

I said, "Why, what's the problem?"

She proceeded to tell me that the patient had presented with a tie-dyed t-shirt and a headset listening to the Grateful Dead. I then again asked, "So, what's the problem?"

She said, "He won't take the headset off."

I said, "So what? Keep moving your lips and he'll get curious." My hygienist proceeded to keep talking.

Sure enough, the patient pulled the headset off and said, "What'd ya say?" This was the point at which she finally had his interest. And that patient not only accepted and treated his periodontal and restorative needs, but also referred his wife, their son, and his sister to my practice. This was the first patient in my practice who didn't bleed post-periodontal therapy. Here was a Case Type III periodontal patient who required no drying agent for subgingival crown margins. I only wish *all* dentists could experience the joy of treating patients like these. Do you know what a pleasure it is to not receive a bloodbath during those preparations?

## Running Your Perio Numbers

Many dentists actually believe they have a vibrant periodontal program in their practice. To properly determine whether this is true, a simple analysis can be used as a barometer to determine just how much periodontal therapy is actually occurring in a given dental practice. Simply print two separate monthly reports: for simplicity's sake, I'll call these Report A and Report B.

- Report A includes all the following codes: 4341, 4342, 4910, and 1110.

- Report B includes codes 4341, 4342, and 4910.

Now, divide the total number of codes from report B by the total number of codes from report A; this will provide your periodontal percentage. A percent level above 60 percent means you are providing an excellent level of periodontal services to your patients, and you are to be congratulated. This result represents 1 to 3 percent of all dental practices.

If your percentage is between 40 to 60 percent, then you are average: better than some, but still substandard. If your percentage is less than 40 percent (the range in which more than 90 percent of all dental practices fall), then your periodontal program is on life support and needs immediate assistance. Dental practices are losing hundreds of thousands of dollars per hygiene chair every year due to a lack of a structured periodontal program.

For years, I have told dentists that, if given a mere twenty minutes to view randomly the progress notes in a dental office's file cabinet,

I could easily add $200,000 per year to that practice's bottom line. It requires no more time than that to identify the lack of periodontal therapy in the practice. There is absolutely nothing comparable to the instantaneous results a properly established and presented periodontal program can have on the quality of care and bottom line of a dental practice.

Eighty percent of all patients who are writing checks for $80–$100 prophys instead should be writing checks for $1,500–$2,200 in order to treat a disease that ultimately is contributing to their own shortened life expectancy.

# 16

# Talking About Wealth—And Health

Discussing wealth in our profession can be a very precarious undertaking. Dentists tend to be very tight-lipped about this subject. I have found dental consultant and speaker Linda Miles's discussion about money to be very compelling. She once said, "Money isn't everything, but it runs a close second to oxygen." Try living without it and then tell me how much it doesn't matter.

I personally think dentists are *extremely* deserving of wealth with no room or regard for guilt. They gave up the best years of their lives to be where they are. For most dentists, the educational journey began somewhere between the ages of seventeen and twenty years old and ended between twenty-five and thirty. Those represent some of the most energetic, enjoyable years of most people's lives; we dentists spent them primarily with our noses in books. In addition to that was the added pressure of competing with the best students for the best grades. I am not implying that those efforts were not worthwhile. I am, however, suggesting that the majority of dentists are throwing away the financial rewards they richly deserve for all of that work. When implemented and presented properly, the structured periodontal program allows you and your staff to work far fewer hours, perform only those procedures that fit your personal comfort zone, and create generational wealth.

Physical duress alone is catastrophic in our profession. If you've experienced none of this (yet), then in all likelihood, you haven't been in practice long enough. Degenerative neck injuries, spinal surgeries, hip and knee replacements, and carpal tunnel casualties tend to pile up as the years go by.

As a result of my own occupational injuries, I do not wish for any dentists to be left unprepared financially if and when such injuries occur. If dentistry is going to abuse the body (and it will), then for the love of God, position yourself financially to live comfortably and without financial burdens. Disability policies are wonderful, but most (unless grandfathered) will expire at the age of sixty-five. Unless you are paying exorbitant premiums, monthly disability payments will not allow you to maintain your current or desired lifestyle.

The ideal lifestyle offers complete financial freedom, and only a handful of dentists ever achieve this. There is a very simple formula to determine your net worth, or rather, more importantly, what that net worth should be. To find your location on the road to financial freedom, simply take your age times your pretax income, then divide that number by ten.

For example, let's assume your pretax income is $140,000. If you are forty years old, then your net worth should be $560,000. If you are fifty years old, it should be $700,000, and if you're sixty years old it should be approximately $840,000. Unfortunately, for most dentists, their net worth is not consistent with their age and income.

Most people believe that as dentists, we should have excessive wealth accumulation, primarily due to our educational status. Strangely enough, the correlation between education and wealth accumulation is *not* linear. Many years of income production are sacrificed to the educational process while debt becomes stockpiled acquiring that coveted education. One of the most troubling reasons for low net worth, however, is the societal pressure to spend excessively which is brought to bear on those with higher educational levels, diminishing the prospect of financial freedom in our profession.

By the age of fifty-five, the average American dentist has accumulated assets of about $250,000 (noninclusive of the value of the home or the dental practice). To determine the net income of the practice, subtract overhead and taxes from gross production. A popular formula for determining the selling price of a dental practice is one and a half times the net practice income. This, added to accumulated assets (about $250,000) needs to result in a number much greater than six digits, because a number of that magnitude invested aggressively (high risk) can be easily lost, and yet if invested passively won't allow sufficient income to sustain the desired lifestyle. In other words, the principal is not sufficient (the net worth is too low), and if you bury it in a mattress, inflation will melt it away like snow on a sunny seventy-degree day.

The purpose of this exercise is to illustrate that your accumulated principal must be sufficient to support you in both good times and bad, and preferably via interest alone. The dentist must earmark certain monies generated on a consistent basis to be used as an investment tool to allow for a substantial portfolio from which you can live handsomely.

## A Perio Program Builds Wealth Without Risk

The investment tool I recommend is not seasonal. Neither does it disappear in tough economic times. That tool is the structured periodontal program and continues to resupply the coffers of that portfolio throughout the life of the dental practice. Periodontal therapy has no boundaries and is the best-kept secret in most dental practices, requiring no new patients to implement; it is always the gift that keeps on giving.

Over the next twenty-five years, the financial core of dentistry will be represented by those forty-five and older. These mouths are not filled with restorative needs, but are indeed swamped in periodontal disease. It is rampant. The hidden, lost, or dormant income in a dental practice is not found in implants, crown and bridge, or orthodontics. Rather, it is found in periodontics and represents additional six-digit income—and the first number of the six-digits is greater than three.

Periodontal therapy in the general practice is *the* system for financial stability—an untapped gold mine in virtually all dental practices that has existed since the shingle was hung out to open the practice. Unless someone mines the gold, then for all practical purposes, it doesn't even exist. The excavator for this gold is the periodontal probe. Simply pick it up, place it in the patient's mouth, and back up the Brinks truck.

Periodontal disease affects 75 to 90 percent of the adult population, yet only 1 to 3 percent of our hygiene services are involved in treating it. I wonder: If there were a 75 to 90 percent incidence of crown and bridge need, would only 1 to 3 percent of our dental services be directed toward treating that? *No way.* Dentists value crown and bridge therapy for a couple of good reasons: it provides a high-quality long-term solution for the patient, and it generates a profit for the dental practice. Currently, neither of these criteria apply to the majority of a dental practice's hygiene department, which are *not* providing high-quality long-term solutions for their patients' periodontal needs, and certainly are *not* generating a significant profit in that hygiene chair. Dentists simply seem to be chasing their tails and looking for love in all the wrong places.

If you were to examine the daysheets (schedules) of the majority of basic, single-hygienist practices, you would find eight to ten prophys per day on the books. Let's suppose the prophy fee is $100, so with ten such patients, the hygienist generates $1,000 per day from prophys. Now let's propose, just for giggles, that two of those ten patients needed and accepted periodontal therapy. That's a 20 percent acceptance rate. Impossible, but just go with me here. The fee per program is $1,500.

At that acceptance and fee rate, you will have generated $3,000 for the two periodontal patients, and that still isn't your total daily production. You receive the $100 for each of the remaining bloody prophys and for both prophys upon completion of your two periodontal therapy patients. Your daily hygiene production just went from $1,000 to $4,000—and how simple was that?

Fortunately, this isn't the full story, because in the worst statistical scenario, *seven of those ten* daily hygiene patients will need and accept periodontal therapy. So, in reality, your daily hygiene production explodes from $1,000 to $11,500.

Even if you were to *inadequately* run this system and only generated $5,000 per day, you still will have increased your hygiene production by a factor of *five times*. These same numbers can be extrapolated to include scenarios of two, three, or more hygienists. Hence, it is very easy to visualize a day in hygiene with multiple hygienists producing $20,000–$40,000 per day with the entire team contributing to the treatment of this disease while providing the highest quality of care for your patients. It is a win-win proposition.

# 17

# The Business Side of Dentistry

In 1987, I was prepping twenty to thirty units of crown and bridge per month. Not bad. Not bad in a town of 1,850 people which, when I first opened my practice, had a dental IQ that was negligible. I used to seat my patients in hygiene and ask them to give me three reasons they had teeth. Few could name as many as two. But in October 1987, I installed the structured periodontal program in the same practice, and for the next four years, I was generating eighty-five to 150 units of crown and bridge per month. Had someone told me this was accomplished in downtown Manhattan, NY, I might still question it, but in the middle of a cornfield in Illinois?

During this time, I actually had a day in which I produced seventeen units of crown and bridge and at the completion of that day, I was found lying on my back in an unequipped treatment room. My hygienist walked by and said, "What's the problem?"

I said, "I'm exhausted."

At that point, my receptionist walked by and said, Well, you might as well get used to it. Tomorrow is no different."

Don't get me wrong; I wasn't complaining, as it was a nice problem to have. It became a benchmark during the first four years of the structured periodontal program: every day I walked in and looked at that day's schedule, I was averaging six to ten units of crown and bridge per day. Do the math and you'll see that was simply astounding. The point of this historical reference is that this occurred *only* after the periodontal program had been installed in the practice, because this structured program rejuvenates and drives the restorative end of the practice.

When a dentist's career begins, he or she is almost universally smothered in an enormous amount of debt: undergraduate education (about $80,000), dental school ($200,000–$400,000), purchasing an existing practice ($250,000–$500,000), building a practice ($600,000), the land to build it on ($100,000–$1,000,000) depending on location, location, location. Equipment costs (chairs; radiographic units; film processor, digital or otherwise; vacuum pump; compression; scanning systems; and cart or wall-mount delivery units; all of this can easily reach $140,000 to $200,000). The utilities, taxes, and maintenance will generally cost $2 to $12 per square foot per year. Interior construction costs are $100 to $140 per square foot, while design and engineering fees are 10 to 14 percent of the total construction costs. These costs lead to a staggering monthly payment, which I believe forces most dental school graduates into corporate dentistry as opposed to owning their own business. The ticket out of the corporate merry-go-round is the structured periodontal program. When properly implemented and presented in a dental practice this system generates massive amounts of revenue above and beyond what that hygienist is already producing, allowing the dental school graduate's ambitions of private practice ownership to be realized.

Unfortunately, the average dentist typically receives only three weeks of any form of business curriculum (which, by the way, is three weeks more than I received as a 1980 graduate of Southern Illinois University School of Dental Medicine. As a result, not surprisingly, in a 2006 survey by the Academy of General Dentistry, the majority of dentists stated that they were overwhelmed as business owners. They also stated that if they had to do it all over again, they would not have chosen a career in dentistry. Surprised? Not me. No, no, *not at all*. The sad thing about all of this is that only *one business decision* is lacking in order to turn this mindset on a dime.

The worst business decision a dentist can make (and most make it) is not informing, diagnosing and treating periodontal disease. The fact that insurance companies are paying more money, more often, to treat this disease makes the decision to treat it even easier.

An average day in hygiene (without a structural periodontal program) includes seven prophys and exams, one gross debridement, four sets of bitewings, and two fluoride treatments. This average day generates about $1,232, or $154 per hour. Now, the question begging to be asked is, "How much of that $154 per hour does it cost the doctor to operate that chair?" The answer? About $95 (62 percent)!

An average day in hygiene with a structured periodontal program includes two prophys and exams, one case Type I patient, three Case

Type II patients, one periodontal maintenance visit, one full-mouth series and exam and one set of vertical bitewings, two sets of basic bitewings, one localized antibiotic, and three fluoride treatments. This day generates $6,139, or $767 per hour.

And what is the cost of operating this chair per hour? Not significantly more than the $95 per hour to operate the hygiene chair in a day *without* periodontal therapy. But just for the fun of it, let's double the overhead. Let's suppose it costs $190 per hour to operate the hygiene chair with the structural periodontal program. Even if this were the case (and it isn't), the next obvious question should be, "Do you want to give up $95 of $154 every hour in hygiene, or would you prefer to give up $190 of $767 each hour in hygiene?" Or look at it this way: You, the doctor, can realize $59 per hour in hygiene, or you can generate $577 each hour in that hygiene chair. Going to have to think about this? *Dear God, I hope not.*

A single hygienist can see sixteen total periodontal patients per month in a hygiene treatment room and generate far more income than seeing 112 prophy patients during the same time. Sixteen periodontal patients at an average fee of $1,350 will generate $21,600 for the month. The 112 prophy patients at a collective fee of $80 each will generate $8,960. This hygienist can see one patient per day for sixteen days and take the rest of each day off with pay, or see four patients per day for four days and take the remaining three weeks off with pay and still more than double his or her monthly production. I can't envision a scenario in which any hygienist would renounce these options.

Here's the reality: the hygienist can see 14 percent of the number of monthly patients and yet still generate two or three times the income. All this, and still doing what's right for every patient. How much better can it get?

## Patient Ability To Pay And Priorities

Despite having written periodically throughout this book about the *financial* benefits of periodontal therapy for the dental practice, it's *not* just about the money. It is actually about what the hygiene department is *not* providing and what hygiene patients are *not* receiving. It is also not about whether patients can afford treatment, but instead about where they want to spend their money.

I am fully aware that we all have some patients who cannot afford anything we do in a dental practice—but that's the exception, not the rule. Many years ago, a patient pulled up to my office in a brand new Mercedes. As she entered the hygiene treatment room, it was obvious she was wearing a pair of designer jeans. If you were to run your finger down the crease, you would have received a severe paper cut. Upon completion of both restorative and periodontal exams and presentations, she said, "Well, I can't afford any of this."

She proceeded to pay her bill at the front desk, and as she walked out of the office, I said to my receptionist, "Shut the practice down."

I was asked, "Why? Where are you going?"

I said, "I'm going to follow her around all day to see where she's spending her money, because she sure isn't giving any of it to dentistry."

Since the majority of our patients *can* afford dental treatment, our job as dental practitioners is to be certain they understand it is far more important to treat a disease that may be shortening their life expectancy than to drive the Mercedes or wear the designer jeans. This particular patient could have done both.

# 18

# My Journey

The year 2014 was a very difficult one for me. I lost my father in July, and subsequent to that, I was speaking to a relatively large group of dentists and staff in Washington, DC. As I was standing at the lectern speaking, I felt my legs "disappear." I had a pretty good idea what was going on, because I'd had other symptoms for years that I had simply ignored. I wasn't about to disrupt my career for any ailment that I could tolerate.

Well, standing at that lectern, I knew if I walked out from behind it as I usually do, I might go straight to the floor. I held on to it for the remainder of the presentation, and when it concluded, I flew home knowing that an appointment with my physician was no longer optional.

After several weeks, I had an appointment at Northwestern Memorial Hospital in Chicago, Illinois. The diagnosis was not a shock. Two lumbar discs were essentially gone, and I needed extensive back surgery. While in the Chicago area for my appointment, I went out for lunch and took a taxi. Upon leaving the restaurant, I had the bright idea to walk back (only three blocks) to the hospital. Things had gotten so bad by that point, I couldn't navigate 100 feet without having to sit on the curb. It required thirty-five minutes for me to walk three blocks.

My surgeon told me that dentistry, genetics, and flying (thirty to forty flights per year) for twenty-five years were contributing factors to the destruction of my back. The surgery was originally scheduled for one day, but on the morning of my surgery, I was advised by the surgeon that the procedure would require five hours the first day through the abdomen and eight hours the second day through my back. All said, I am today the proud owner of two eight-inch rods, ten two-inch screws, and a cage in my back. To add insult to injury, I developed post-op neuropathy. This resulted in foot pain at all times, so to help alleviate this, in 2016 I had a neurostimulator placed in my back to help "disguise" the pain.

My recovery, or rehabilitation, took about two years. During this time, I was able to derive answers to a question that had always bewildered me. I couldn't understand why some dental offices that had implemented the periodontal program would show a leveling off of their success over a period of time. This had never been a problem in my practice, and I wondered what caused these variations. The answer, it turns out, is two-fold. First, the structured periodontal program cannot be customized during a seminar, because every dental office has its own comfort zone, and if that comfort zone is disrupted, it really doesn't matter what you are attempting to implement—it simply won't be sustainable. The other reason for variations in the success of the program over time is staff turnover. All systems (unless engaged by all staff members) tend to be disrupted by selective staff turnover. Herein lies the reason that I have dedicated my future to providing seminars, consulting, podcasts, webinars, and online continuing education (CE) training courses. My objective is to do whatever it takes to get this critical message into the normal routine of all dental practices.

Let me share my journey. I didn't come from a poor family, but I did come from the lower half of the middle class. My father was a plasterer by trade and also worked at the Chrysler Corporation in Belvidere, Illinois.

When I was five years old, I fell in a freshly combined cornfield and drove a cornstalk through the center of my right eye. I was told that, had it entered any other way, I would be blind in that eye. I took large doses of penicillin and I wore a black patch over my eye for several weeks. The amazing thing is that today I'm sixty-three years old and still don't have the need for glasses.

At seventeen, I had two bad health experiences. In the same year, my appendix ruptured, and I inadvertently cut my right wrist open with a porcelain ladle as it broke in half as I was doing dishes. I had to take notes with my left hand for six weeks. I tried to use that as a reason to never hand-wash a dish again. The cut caused me to lose most of the feeling on the top of my right thumb. The surgeon asked me what I was going to do for a career, and I said I wanted to be a dentist. He told me that, had the injury been placed one sixtieth of an inch differently, that would have been only a pipe dream.

In April 1967, a brutal category four tornado destroyed about 25 percent of our community. The wind speeds were prolific, and the storm wiped out our local high school. Many people were severely injured or died in this disaster, and the high school gymnasium was used temporarily as a morgue for some of the lost students. I was twelve years old at the time, in Confirmation class at Zion Lutheran Church.

There were no warnings or sirens to caution the community about what was about to occur. My recollection is leaving the church in the late afternoon and seeing the green-black sky. I was so nervous, I just started running home (about ten blocks in distance). As I ran, I found myself jumping over downed electrical wires; the wind was unlike any I had ever experienced. I looked into the sky and observed telephone poles that looked like javelins in the air and houses without roofs. As I ran by a tree near the high school area of town, I observed a piece of straw that had entered the south side of a tree (diameter about two feet) and what appeared to be the same piece of straw exiting the north side of that tree. To this day, I'm not sure how that is even possible, but there it was.

Kids had buried themselves in the dirt of an open field in order to avoid the debris flying through the air. School buses had been flipped like toys. I kept running as fast as I could until I got home, wondering all the way if our house was still standing. Our home was fine, except for some roof damage, but the town itself was declared a disaster area and took years to recover. My farther had owned a home, which he rented out, and the upstairs apartment was left with no roof, open to the sky. A couple of days later, in April, a snow storm dumped four to six inches of snow into this apartment. My dad and I spent a full day shoveling snow over the walls and down to the ground below.

What was many people's disaster became, for some, an opportunity. My father was always very good with respect to carpentry, plastering, roofing, etc. The community at that time was in need of as many carpenters as it could find, and my father made the decision to leave the security of Chrysler Corporation and venture out on his own, with Robert L. Tripke Remodeling and Repair. He made the correct decision; he was happier doing what he loved and became more successful than he had ever hoped. He once told me that he didn't want to depend on any job, such as Chrysler, to dictate his opportunities to provide or succeed. This was sage advice which returned to me in spades years later, when he said there was much more responsibility but also freedom in being your own boss. I never forgot that.

My father always had me working on jobs with him. One of which comes to mind is the day I mixed plaster in a basement and carried it up two flights of outdoor stairs during the winter. I couldn't carry five-gallon pails, as I was too small, so my dad had me carry plaster in plastic ice cream buckets. This day started at 7:00 a.m. and ended at 7:00 p.m. When I got home, I went upstairs to take a bath and I never returned for dinner as I passed out exhausted on my bed. Shortly after this I decided there had to be easier ways to make a living, so I started charging my sisters to use the bathroom: maybe not the nicest thing to do, but you'd be surprised how much people would pay if they had to go *that badly*.

I also grew up a huge sports fan and my dad built a basketball backboard and rim on the roof of our garage. The first morning it was completed, I went outside (about fifty degrees Fahrenheit) and shot baskets from 7:00 a.m. to 10:00 p.m. I guess you could safely say I was by then obviously diagnosed as OCD. (I have always been a stickler for detail. At the age of eight, I became obsessed with having a perfectly clean yard. I once raked it so often that I eliminated the grass.) In high school, I was fortunate to be one of twelve players on the school basketball team in a class of about 380 students. I ran cross-country for four years (hated to run) because the cross-country coach was also the basketball coach. If you wanted to play basketball, then you also either ran or were on the football team. I was the "runt of the litter" in basketball, but I always tried to outwork the others to allow myself the privilege of being on that team.

When I graduated from high school, I was voted one of two students "least likely to succeed." I'm sure that was a gag, but nonetheless, I never forgot it. In 1972, after high school, I was signed, sealed, and essentially delivered to Illinois State University (ISU), where my major was physical education, not pre-dental. I always felt sports was my logical direction in life, but I was torn at that time, because I knew there were three things I wanted in life, and they weren't going to happen in coaching. My three desires were self-employment, working with my hands (not outside, though), and financial independence. I really couldn't see how coaching was going to allow me to reach all of those goals. I also knew that, from the time I first observed dentistry, it fascinated me, and it would give me an opportunity to meet all three criteria for a career choice.

At this time in my life, I was also struggling with the question my father always asked me each time we would finish a job: "Do you want to make your living with your back or with your head?" I chose to make my living with my head, but ultimately destroyed my back doing so. (The irony of how that question would work itself out in my life is priceless.) I was seventeen years old, just out of high school, and literally tormenting myself to make a life changing decision. I recall being in the basement of my parent's home during this time, and this so-called life choice was weighing so heavily on me that, listening to "Father and Son" by Cat Stevens, out of total frustration, I drove my fist into one of my dad's plastered walls. Plaster, for those of you who are only familiar with the drywall world, is *extremely* difficult to break, and this was sand-finished plaster, so not only didn't the wall break, it also took the skin (several layers) off three knuckles. I *still* don't know why I didn't break my hand or fingers. At the point of that frustration, I knew what I was going to do, but had several reasons to believe I wouldn't make it into dentistry. One reason: I had zero science background in high school. Another: I was extremely worried about the cost of the journey.

On that day, I dropped out of my commitment to ISU and enrolled at a local junior college (Rock Valley Junior College). This decision would allow me to sign up for the proper curriculum and receive my first two years of college education at far less cost. The irony is I would ultimately end up practicing dentistry just twenty-seven minutes from ISU. I thought my father would be thrilled because I was saving so much money, but he was upset and seemed embarrassed. His view was that a junior college was not the way to get a good education, and

I think he felt that his friends would look down at him, because his son was attending a lower class of higher education. Years later, he confessed that this was precisely how he had felt, but admitted I had made the correct decision.

I started by taking a chemistry course, among others, that I was not qualified for. This was Chemistry 101, and if you had little or no experience in this subject (I had none) you belonged in Chemistry 100 (which offered no college credit, but was an appropriate course for my experience level). Well, I wasn't going to consider wasting an entire semester on a course for zero credits. I dove into the course, studied ten to twelve hours per day, and on my first exam, I received a D+. This one about did me in. I went home, sat on the porch, and when my dad came home, he wanted to know what was bothering me. I told him what had happened, and he said, "Well, maybe you'd better try something else."

This was like holding the cross up to Dracula.

My father's reply so angered me that I was devastated. Looking back, I could have responded two ways: Throw in the towel and quit, because I had given it my best effort, or dig my heels in deeper and push through this. Several years later, when my dad was dying, I told him that those words were the driving force for all my success. He said "Really?" I told him I was so angry at those words that nothing was going to stop me. I rallied and refocused my study habits, spending more time studying the *right* information versus spending too much time studying *too much* information.

I earned three Bs that first semester, and I knew the three Bs were not going to get me into dental school. It had to be As across the board. From that day forward, I earned a 4.0 throughout my undergraduate education at Rock Valley Junior College and Southern Illinois University. It was in 1975 that I was accepted into SIU-Carbondale, where I attended for two years. I took my first Dental Admissions Test (DAT) at the completion of my first semester at SIU, and the experience taught me that I wasn't ready for dental school. I needed *many* more courses under my belt to successfully navigate the DAT exam. I proceeded to take human anatomy, cell physiology, and mammalian physiology, among others, to prepare myself. The mammalian physiology course tested multiple (five to ten) chapters per exam and all exams were short essay (fifty questions) from 7:00 p.m.–9:00 p.m. in the evening. That one course taught me *I could beat all the odds*. My major was physiology, while my minor was nutrition. My second DAT included a reading comprehension section that was fifty questions about nutrition, so you might say that I was blessed that day (never read it, but answered all fifty questions).

In Carbondale, I lived in a trailer off campus for two years. The trailers were about twenty feet apart, and my neighbor used to open his door and sit outside in his underwear playing his guitar. Music blared, cats ran in and out of his trailer, and I stuffed cotton in my ears to try to focus. Despite these distractions, I went on to obtain my bachelor's degree in physiology and completed my undergraduate level of education with a grade point average of 3.89. I knew this was the time to pursue my dental school application. On March 28, 1977, I received a certified letter delivered to my trailer, and I was certain that the dental school would not waste a certified letter just to inform me that I had been turned down. It was, indeed, the motherlode; I had been accepted to Southern Illinois University School of Dental Medicine, the last of a three-year dental program, later to become my two-and-a-half-year journey.

Dental school was equally challenging and stressful, but in a different way. The actual letter grades weren't as relevant, because after all, whether you received an A- or a B+, you're still Doctor Jones, right? Dental school's lessons were more about dealing with rejection, which is highly relevant in private practice. I sincerely feel that the largest obstacle to gaining financial freedom in dentistry is the issue of rejection. That, and giving dentistry away (I'm not referring to charity). By the time dentists graduate from dental school, they have been indoctrinated with rejection. During dental school, you learn very quickly that regardless of what you do, it's seldom "good enough." It was well known in school that the best response from an instructor was *no response at all*. The problem this creates in our profession is that by the time you leave dental school, you will do anything in your power to avoid rejection. This includes, of course, not properly presenting treatment plans with the confidence that patients will accept them. Personally, the high acceptance of periodontal treatment plans is what removed my fear of rejection. An employee of mine once said to me, referring to periodontal therapy, "If you do this in Chenoa, they will run you out of here on a rail."

I responded, "There could be worse things than having to leave Chenoa," and it was never going to happen anyway. It's all about telling the truth to the patient and about the proper presentation to the patient.

In the fall of 1979, I was standing in line to pay tuition in dental school and began a discussion with two other students about early graduation. This was intriguing to me for many obvious reasons— money, the final end to an eight-year stint in school, and getting an early jump on private practice, among others. But it also scared the hell out of me. I had quite a bit to yet accomplish, so the prospect of early graduation was quite an undertaking. It was October, and I had to cram all my remaining graduation requirements into about two-and-a-half months as opposed to finishing them in the allotted eight to nine months. Well, I can assure you I was hellbent to get out of the rejection carousel and finally make a living and begin to service some of my debt.

This two-and-a-half-month journey was exhausting, as our mock boards had been moved up to be taken earlier at the school and we would have to take our Northeast Regional board exams at Loyola University in Chicago. This meant lining up board patients and travel arrangements, including hotels, not to mention meals. After my first day taking clinical boards in Chicago, I returned to my hotel room, completely drained, only to find that my room had been robbed. I lost all my cash and a watch, but still had a great day, as I had prepped and fabricated the best inlay of my short dental career—a beveled margin on the gingival floor of that box prep that only a dentist could appreciate. After the clinicals and the written boards, I climbed in my car and drove back to Alton, Illinois (home of SIU-SDM), about a five-

and-a-half-hour trip. When I walked into my basement apartment, I fell on the bed and slept for sixteen hours.

I proceeded to get what felt like the bubonic plague, and I was sick in bed for two weeks. It was just the crash that occurs after an incredible forced high that had lasted almost three-and-a-half months, start to finish. I lived in that apartment and waited for almost two months to receive my verdict: two agonizing months just to see if I had passed. I have never understood why it takes such a long period of time to grade and notify students of such a large accomplishment in their life.

In the spring of 1980, I officially became a dentist and acted upon a contact I had received in dental school. I had heard of a small town in central Illinois that was looking for a dentist and I had previously contacted the community. The name of the town was Chenoa. I drove there to meet and speak with community officials about the possible opportunity to be their dentist (their previous dentist had retired). I knew that if I were to set up as the only dentist in a town of 1,850 people, I could build that practice in about one to two years, versus the five to ten years it might require to become established in a larger, metropolitan area, and I wasn't wrong. I have been advised by dental practice brokers that the millennials of our population of dentists have no interest in small communities, which I would say is probably their biggest mistake. I, too, had to choose between lifestyle and income. Going into practice in Chenoa was the *first* best business decision I ever made. Smaller communities are goldmines in dentistry. The cost of living is much less, and the growth and development of a dental practice is light-years faster.

I started out in Chenoa in a temporary dental facility which my father and his friend helped me to construct inside an existing dilapidated building. The office was about 500 square feet: no private office, no lab, no ceiling, no doors—wide open. I had a bell tied to a string on an outside glass door. If I heard the bell jingle, I knew someone was coming in, and so I stood up in the reception room and said, "Hi, I'm Dr. Tripke," as I shook hands and took the patient back to be seated. My receptionist's area was three feet by four feet, triangular, and in there was a four-drawer vertical file. My biggest problem in this office was finding someone small enough to work behind that front desk, because regardless of how skinny you were, you had to turn sideways to get in and out.

This was 1980, the economy was horrific, and prime interest rates hovered around 21 percent. I felt like leaving dental school was like jumping out of the frying pan just to get into the fire. Unemployment was also very high, and after working for about six months, I felt I needed to do something to make my business more appealing to attract customers. People certainly didn't want to leave work (lose pay) to visit the dentist. I decided to work day and evening hours.

I worked Monday and Wednesday, 10:00 a.m. to 7:00 p.m., and Tuesdays and Thursdays, 8:00 a.m. to 7:00 p.m.. I also worked Fridays, 8:00 a.m. to 5:00 p.m. and Saturdays 8:00 a.m. to noon. Availability was the key. Regardless of how much downtime I had, I was available to patients early, worked over their lunch hours, and in the evenings for those who couldn't or wouldn't leave work. *And it worked.*

My business was growing quickly. I grossed $110,000 in the first nine months of practice. That may not seem like a lot today, but my banker says it would have been about $275,000 in today's dollars. I'll take it. My rent was $110 per month (and I paid no utilities). After about fourteen months, I decided to take a leap of faith and sign on to build my own dental facility (all brick, 2,600 square feet, four ops, a private office, twelve-seat reception room, kitchen, and an attached garage). This and the home I had purchased set me back about $550,000. My office loan was through the Bank of Chenoa via Industrial Revenue Bonds, which I thought were a steal at 13.75 percent. My home loan was 13 percent. My office payments were required to be made in two yearly installments; one payment was $15,000 principal, and the other (six months later) was $10,000 in interest. These were exorbitantly high payments which required discipline to save money. My stress levels were very high, and I was working long hours, so I am thankful that, at the time, I had no children, because if I had, I'm sure that I would have only rarely seen them. I lived this life for seven years, taking no vacations, no time off, making myself available twenty-four hours a day to my patients. But as my father always said, "Hard work pays off." Right again!

# 19

# Working Longer Is Not The Answer

S adly, most dentists believe that in order to generate more income for the practice, everyone needs to treat a high volume of patients and work long hours. This is not only wrong, but is also the recipe for a shortened career in dentistry.

Look, for example, at the predictable profit generation of the structured periodontal program. Consider for a moment that the net income from a single hygiene chair, on the low end, is about $150 per hour with this system in place. With this in mind, it is easy to see how dentists can generate a mere $100 per hour in their restorative chairs and still reach all of their necessary financial goals. The $100 per hour translates to one crown per day (at $1,000 per unit). At that point, relax in your private office listening to your favorite radio station and simply wait for the hygienist to notify you of the need for an exam.

As can be seen, this removes an enormous amount of pressure in the dental practice regarding business and production goals. If another highly productive procedure were to cancel on that same day, *no worries.* The hygiene department will continue to carry the day from a production standpoint.

I can't stress enough: In addition to the dramatically enhanced quality of care being provided, the purpose of all this is to work far less and generate far more income. If that isn't appealing to you, then you might want to see a physician.

The structured periodontal program is a team effort and will not operate at peak efficiency without a total team approach. In other words, it cannot operate with only the doctor and hygienist on board—at least, not nearly as effectively and productively.

In 1987, my hygiene department (one hygienist) was generating $4,000 to $5,000 a month—our hygiene department produced $56,000 that year with no periodontal program. In 1988, the same hygienist, using the structured program, generated $221,000. In 2018 dollars, that translates to $468,000 per year with one hygienist managing the program. In 1987, my practice produced $400,000 without the structured periodontal program. In 1988, with the program, the practice produced $950,000 with the same doctor and hygienist utilizing the system.

Looking at the math, it's obvious: the restorative dentistry *also* jumped—from about $350,000 in 1987 to about $700,000 in 1988. This amazing revelation occurred because periodontal therapy accelerates restorative in a prolific manner. The $950,000 production in 1988 translates to $2,014,000 in 2018 numbers.

The real kicker here? We worked far less, saw fewer patients, provided a much higher quality of care and more than doubled the practice's production. I was only performing procedures within my comfort zone, no longer feeling obligated to treat every dental problem that walked in the door. The pressure was off, and I was for the first time in my life enjoying *every moment* in that practice.

Who doesn't want to work less and make far more income? Ask dentists if they would prefer to see half the patients and generate two to four times the income. I can assure you, you'll get a resounding "Yes!"

In October 1987, I was $550,000 in debt. In November of 1989, three days before Veteran's Day, I walked into the Bank of Chenoa and cut the last check on that debt. During the first two years (1987–1989) of implementing this system in my dental practice, I retired *all* of my debt—the equivalent in 2018 dollars of retiring $1,600,000 in two years. How many dentists ever graduated from dental school and even dreamed of being debt free inside of five years? *Not one.* Thirty-five years is probably a stretch.

There is no way possible for that to have happened for me without the structured periodontal program. In all likelihood, I might still be picking you-know-what with the chickens.

# 20

# My Final Dirty Little Secret: You Ain't Getting Younger

Here's the point of this entire book. Restorative levels are down, stress levels are up, production is down, liability is up, and my final dirty little secret, doctor, is that you ain't getting any younger.

There are three rewarding goals in dentistry: Save teeth, improve smiles, and extend lives. Only one procedure accomplishes all three. You don't have to be the best dentist to be financially successful in dentistry, but you do have to have the proper system in place, or you haven't even got a chance.

When my dental career began in Chenoa, I was in a temporary facility. I was supposed to be there for two months, but I was in there for two years. The facility by itself was grounds for leaving dentistry. I didn't sleep in a bed for two years. I couldn't sleep. Rather, I laid in a recliner in front of a TV set every night.

I once had a man come into the office wanting an extraction, so I seated him, gave the anesthetic, and proceeded to extract the tooth. He walked to the front desk and said, "Can I give you five bucks for that today?" I answered, "Give it to me. It's five more than I had yesterday."

Long story short, that man walked out of my office and across the street into a tavern. How did I know? I was sitting in the reception area looking out the window, as I had no other patients. Twenty-five minutes later, the man came out of the tavern. How did I know that? Because I was still sitting there. I had no other patients.

He walked out of the tavern, stumbling down the street with a twelve-pack of Stroh's beer under each arm.

Now, let's ask a couple of questions. Did the man spend more than five bucks on two twelve-packs? Did the man spend more than five bucks in order to get that drunk? Of course. So, there's only one more question to ask: who is the moron? Well, it's obviously me. I took the man out of pain and received five bucks. The tavern got him drunk and got paid. From that point on, my motto was, "If you are going to pay me half the money to extract the tooth, then I'm taking it half-way out of the socket, and I promise it will feel different than when you came in. When you return with the rest of the money, I will finish the job." (I'm sure you feel the jesting, but no: the horse only gets to kick me once. I never go back for the second time.)

I'm in my new office, and had no idea anyone was in the operatory, and I heard a voice that said, "Nothing makes me madder."

So I stick my head in the room and said, "Than what?, I don't even know who you are."

The man looked at me and said, "I come in here, you pull a tooth, you charge me $150, and it doesn't take you five minutes."

So, I looked at him and said, "If it will make you feel better, I'll take longer! I'll do a little wiggle and take a walk, do a little wiggle and take a walk and do a little wiggle and take a walk. I can drag this out for an hour if it makes you feel better."

Well he didn't get it. So, I looked at him and said, "You didn't pay me for taking the tooth out in five minutes. You paid me because I didn't take your eyeball with it." In other words, he was paying me for the education that I paid for.

He *still* didn't get it.

Now, I knew what I was about to do with this man, and I couldn't stop laughing inside. I said, "I'll tell you what we can do. I will have you get yourself numb. I will have you lay a syringe tip under your lip. When I tell you, I want you to wiggle your lip. Next, I will give you a timed command. When I say this, I want you to shove it."

I said, "If you think that felt good, wait till we get to the roof of your mouth. The next thing I will do is give you something that looks like a screwdriver, and when I give you the word, I want you to place it next to the tooth and turn it. Next, I will give you something that looks like a pair of pliers. When I tell you, I want you to grab the tooth and swing to the right, swing to the left."

I said, "Do you know what is going to happen here? You are going to snap the tooth off at the gumline. This means I'm going to have to cut the tooth out of the bone, and that's going to take a long, long, time ... and isn't that what you're here for?"

Some days, I felt that every wacko in the world would find my practice.

A closing thought: the periodontal program has little bling and it's probably not sexy, but it is the most sustainable, cost-effective, and highly productive entity that can be implemented in a dental practice, today or at any other time. In the end, I can merely ask you to ask yourself a question: It takes five to six minutes to probe a dental patient. So, is that worth increasing hygiene's production by $200–$400 per hour?

I implore dentists *not* to put their heads in the sand with respect to this system, because *this is your gamechanger.* You will only get one or two of these in your lifetime. If you turn your head and ignore it, it doesn't come around again. Please do not waste it.

# APPENDIX A
# Acknowledgments

Tiffany: I need to start by giving thanks to my beautiful wife, soulmate, and best friend, who helped me restart my life and was solely responsible for lifting me up (literally) and kept pushing me forward to chase my dream and my passion, which is speaking and teaching about periodontal therapy for all dentists.

My children, Alex and Brielle: My daily inspiration comes from watching my son and daughter pursue their dreams, and they are both truly amazing, accomplished, and driven young adults. I could not be prouder.

Bill Evans: My mentor, father figure, and the most intelligent man I have ever known. Bill took a chance on me and believed in me before I believed in myself. Without Bill, there would never have been a speaking career.

Vanessa Emerson: My missing link to the restart of my speaking career and an amazing human being who literally helped revive my speaking career. Without her Jumpstart 2018 meeting, I would never have connected with Mark LeBlanc.

Mark LeBlanc: My book shepherd, mentor, and good friend who started it all by saying the first time we met: "You've got a story to tell;

you need to write a book." The ultimate guidance counselor in the uncharted waters of writing a book.

Henry DeVries: My book editor at Indie Books International who eloquently organized and parlayed my thoughts into the book they have become.

Doug Billings: The man who came to know me at the age of thirty-two and traveled across the country representing the company, ProDentec, for which I spoke for almost twenty years. Doug has always been a sounding board, much-needed critic, and a friend I can trust through the ups and downs of providing as many as forty seminars per year. A true confidant.

Doug Billings, David Simpson, Gerry McAnulty, David Cooper, and Chuck Tipton: My Five Amigos and traveling partners for more than two decades. Truer friends were never found, and our life experiences together were priceless.

Scott Bradshaw: The man and friend responsible for curbing my enthusiasm, which at times was over the top.

I must mention all the dentists nationwide who continued to inspire me with their success stories, letters, phone calls, text messages, and emails about how I was able to positively impact their lives. Little did they know, every one of them powerfully impacted my life as well.

And of course, all of my employees over the years who worked so hard to achieve the levels of success with our patients and the practice.

# APPENDIX B
# About the Author

Robert A. Tripke, DMD, implemented an organized approach to nonsurgical periodontal therapy in his Chenoa, Illinois, practice in 1987. Due to the marked elevation in standard of care for his patients as well as a huge positive financial impact on his practice, shortly thereafter he began educating general dentists in these methods and protocols.

For nearly thirty years, Dr. Tripke has provided structured periodontal therapy training with the newest, most effective techniques available. His program is recognized in the industry as the pinnacle of soft-tissue management.

A passionate, animated, and empowering speaker, Dr. Tripke's educational programs have influenced thousands of general dental practices by enhancing the quality of care and dramatically altering the economic status of those practices. In recognition of his successes, Dr. Tripke was featured in the *Dentistry Today* article, "My Unparalleled Success with Soft Tissue Management in a Small Mid-American Town."

Dr. Tripke can be reached at 309-838-8518 or robert@roberttripke.com.

# APPENDIX C
# Patient and Practitioner Q&As: *Guidelines for Conversation*

These verbal conversation prompts are useful and are dialogue guides for conversations with patients who do not readily accept diagnosis and treatment. The most common patient questions and objections are in bold, with recommended responses following. These responses can come from either the hygienist or the dentist.

## X-Rays

**Do you think all those X-rays are necessary?**

This full mouth series of films shows not only your back teeth, but your front ones as well. In the past, films taken on the back teeth were thought to provide enough information about cavities and periodontal disease. Now we know from experience with other patients and the latest research that a great deal more is needed and that without this data you can actually do yourself more harm.

**But isn't that a lot of radiation that is not supposed to be good for you?**

As I mentioned before, if you were to have an abscess or cancerous lesion, we would not be able to know or inform you that it was there if we did not have the films to show us. Leaving that kind of problem in the body will do you far greater harm than this radiation will.

**These films are expensive.**

These films will be able to show us decay in the beginning stages, especially in between the teeth, as well as any bone loss. If we rely on a visual exam alone, often the cavities and bone loss are much greater before they are seen and can be treated. This could mean the difference between a simple filling and a cleaning or a root canal, crown and periodontal surgery. It's your choice.

# Periodontal Exam

*To Help Hygienists Set the Stage for the Exam*

After the full-mouth series of films is taken, I will be doing a periodontal examination in conjunction with the doctor's exam for cavities. This exam is to check to see how healthy the gums and bone around your teeth are, not necessarily the teeth themselves. It will take me only a few minutes to do this exam and it is painless. I will be using a blunt-ended instrument that measures your gums just like a ruler (show probe). When I call out these measurements, we hope to hear numbers like 1, 2, 3. That tells you and me that you are doing well brushing and flossing. Anything greater than 3 means that the gum is pulling away from the teeth and is no longer supporting it. For this reason, there must be infection in those sites and are areas of concern.

**With all this time being taken up by x-rays and exams, will I get my teeth cleaned today?**

If you have a healthy/good perio exam, then yes, I will be doing a routine cleaning today. However, if there are areas in your mouth where you have infection and possible bone loss, it is my hope that you will want to learn of these areas and how to treat them and it may require something more than just a cleaning.

Bleeding is also a sign of infection so I'm going to give you a mirror and together we will determine how you are doing. Have you noticed any bleeding when you're brushing or flossing at home?

**No, I never have any bleeding when I'm brushing; sometimes when I floss, but that's because I floss too hard and cut my gum.**

*(Probing in patient's mouth)*

See the bleeding in this area?

**Well, it never bleeds when I brush. It must be because you're poking with that instrument.**

If I were to touch your hand with this instrument with the same amount of pressure and it were to bleed, would you be concerned? Bleeding in the mouth is no different and is just as much of a concern for us.

**What do those 4s and 5s mean?**

Let me show you in the chart I have here (Periodontal Stages Chart). Let's see. You had 4s, 5s, bleeding, and your tissue is red and puffy. I'll hold your x-rays here too. Can you see in this picture how the probe slides down the tooth and how the gum has pulled away? This is known as periodontal disease. If I were to give you a cleaning, which we do for healthy gums, I would actually be unable to get the infection out. Four and five millimeters down is where your calculus/tartar is.

**So you will not be cleaning my teeth today?**

No, as I stated earlier, I was fully prepared to do a regular cleaning for you. However, after finding these areas of infection, I also wanted you to be aware of them so you could make a decision on treatment. That is why I took the extra time with you today. Since we are going to do the periodontal therapy, we will need to schedule you immediately. If you have any questions, please do not hesitate to contact us. Thank you.

# Other Topics

**My insurance is only going to pay 50 percent, so I am not going to do this treatment.**

I would hope that your health decisions are not all based on insurance benefits. If you broke your arm, would you refuse to have the doctor set it because your insurance would not cover the full amount?

**All this sounds like a lot of work. Can't we just pull 'em?**

"Pulling teeth will leave you with only about thirty pounds per square inch of chewing force, whereas chewing with all your natural teeth is about 300 pounds. Also, there are multiple visits for extractions and a healing phase before placing the dentures and the fee for these procedures exceeds even the periodontal therapy.

**I came here to get my teeth cleaned, and that's what I would like to have done.**

At your request, I will provide you with a cleaning today as long as you are aware that I am leaving tartar below the gumline and the infection may continue.

**You're not going to get all of the tartar? You're going to leave it there?**

Asking me to remove all the tartar requires the time/procedures I spoke of earlier. Anything less is like asking a surgeon to remove half a tumor in half the time he needs; unfortunately, he compromises himself and leaves the other half in the body to carry on further destruction.

**I guess you have to tell me more about this periodontal therapy. I don't want to lose my teeth. Is this new information? Why did you not take these films and do this exam six months ago?**

In the past, emphasis was placed on the control of dental decay. So study and research focused on fluoride and dental sealants and those were introduced. Now with these advances, decay is down by 50 percent. More patients are losing their teeth to periodontal disease than dental decay and because studies have intensified in the area of periodontal disease, more and more information is being sent to us on a daily basis on how to best treat and overcome this disease. The dental field makes advances in research just as the medical profession does on, for instance, lowering cholesterol rates and eating oat bran, etc.

**So, what do we have to do? How many visits, etc.?**

We (doctor and hygienist together) have determined that treatment for this disease will require four visits of about one hour (six teeth per quad x ten minutes per tooth). A visit of about thirty minutes a week later will be the time that we polish and floss your teeth and, more importantly, remeasure or re-probe these areas to see if the gum has re-attached. Remember, we cannot replace the bone you've lost, but we can prevent it from deteriorating any further.

**How many times do I have to go through this?**

As many times as you want to, and hopefully you'll answer that by saying once, which is how many times I want to do this. The reason you have disease is because you haven't been able to remove all the plaque from your mouth, and that hardens into tartar. After you complete the periodontal therapy program, we will place you on a perio maintenance regimen, where we can closely monitor your gums and help prevent you from getting to this point again.

**What does all this cost? I don't have dental insurance, so is this going to be expensive?**

The entire fee for this program, which includes all visits, is $XXX.00. Patients usually pay so much each visit or so much monthly, depending on what they feel comfortable with. I will provide you with a treatment estimate form on your way out today which lists all treatment, including the doctor's restorative care. It is better to schedule for this program as soon as possible so that it does not progress any further. Could you possibly schedule next week?

**I don't know. It sounds pretty expensive to me.**

Well, you have twenty-five teeth, and with this fee that comes to about $15 dollars per tooth. You have more than that invested in those fillings and crowns you have, and without this treatment you may eventually lose these teeth and any future investment you put in them.

**It doesn't look like I have much choice. I want to keep my teeth, so I'll need to do this.**

I will need your signature stating that you have made your choice and that you are aware that you have periodontal disease and understand everything I've told you. We will also make a copy of this for you to keep for your records if you'd like. Do you have any questions, or is there anything you do not understand? I realize this is a lot of information.

**I have tartar under the gums?**

Tartar under the gums is a lot like getting a splinter under your skin. If you don't remove it, it will fester and cause infection. In a regular cleaning there is no "splinter" for me to remove, because the gums have not pulled away from the tooth and migrated down the root surface. To get the tartar off the root surface I have to do a procedure called root planing (or smoothing of the root) and often it requires anesthesia and a greater amount of time—usually five to ten minutes per tooth.

**Am I going to be sore from this? It sounds awful.**

Once the anesthesia has worn off you can eat and drink normally. For any tenderness you may have to rinse with warm salt water. This is *not* surgery. I will not be pulling the gum away from the tooth or doing any stitches. Patients often tell me their mouths feel better.

**Why didn't you tell me this six months ago? I had a cleaning and you told me everything was fine.**

We have been monitoring your periodontal condition for quite some time. Unfortunately, we have recently noticed that you are taking three steps forward and four steps back. We are, in fact, losing ground in our attempt to control this disease. We have spent an extensive amount of time involved in continuing education regarding the proper sequence and technique to properly treat this disease. In order to properly diagnose the disease, we need a full-mouth set of films to show the bone support for your teeth, and we need six measurements with a periodontal ruler around each tooth to properly diagnose and treatment plan your periodontal condition. Without this information today, it is very likely that the disease will continue to progress and eventually end in tooth loss.

Made in the USA
San Bernardino, CA
07 April 2019